Problem-centred Learning

The Modified Essay Question in Medical Education:
A Handbook for Students, Teachers and Trainers.

Keith Hodgkin, B.M., B.Ch., F.R.C.G.P. F.R.C.P.
Professor of General Practice, Memorial University,
Newfoundland, Canada.

J. D. E. Knox, M.D.(Edin.), F.R.C.P.(Edin.), F.R.C.G.P.
Professor of General Practice, University of Dundee.

Foreword by
Lord Hunt of Fawley, C.B.E., M.A., D.M.Oxon., F.R.C.P., F.R.C.S.
F.R.C.G.P., F.R.A.C.G.P.

Churchill Livingstone
EDINBURGH LONDON AND NEW YORK 1975

CHURCHILL LIVINGSTONE

Medical Division of Longman Group Limited
Distributed in the United States of America by Longman Inc.,
New York and by associated companies, branches and
representatives throughout the world.

ISBN 0 443 01296 2

Library of Congress Cataloging in Publication Data

Hodgkin, Keith.
    Problem centred learning.

    Bibliography: p.
    Includes index.
    1. Medicine--Study and teaching.   2. Medicine--
Problems, exercises, etc.   3. Graduate medical education.
I. Knox, James D.E.   II. Title.
R834.H6   610'.76   75-8587

Printed in Great Britain

Foreword

The authors of this book have spent much time and thought, and have taken a great deal of trouble, in developing the modern examination technique of modified essay questions and in adapting them to the assessment of the professional competence of family doctors.

The young College of General Practitioners nearly decided, at a well-attended general meeting on 21st November, 1959, when it was seven years old, to introduce the passing of an examination as one of the criteria for its membership. The motion was agreed by 112 votes to 44 but, as this was just short of the ¾ majority required for a special resolution, it was not carried. Two years later it was passed with only 15 votes against.

Immediately after this, the subject was brought glaringly before the eyes of the whole profession when a mammoth discussion took place, in the correspondence columns of the *British Medical Journal*, as to whether or not it was possible to assess the work of general practitioners in such a way and, if so, what kind of examination should it be? More than fifty letters appeared during the next few months, leading articles were written, even the lay press became involved, people from many other branches of the profession joined the fray, feelings ran high and, in the end, some of the letters were so fierce that the editor closed the correspondence.

However, those who believed that some kind of test for membership of the College was essential, if its academic standing was to be raised above that of a medical society, had made their point the hard way. In November 1965 the first optional examination was held at the headquarters of the College, with five candidates, four of whom passed. Since then, different techniques have been tried and developed. Last year (1974) 555 candidates sat the examination which is now compulsory; of these 413 passed. Modified essay questions are now an important constituent of it. The fact that we did have an examination for membership played a major part, I am sure, in the decision to grant us our Royal Charter.

This excellent book by Professor Keith Hodgkin and Professor J.D.E. Knox on *Problem-Centred Learning* is full of interesting detail. It should be useful to all who are concerned with

medical education in every branch of our profession -
students, teachers and examiners - especially to those
who hope to be or already are family doctors, and to
those who teach and test them in the knowledge and
reactions they will need in the real-life situations
which they will meet over the years in any good general
practice.

1975   *Hunt of Fawley,*
                        Past President,
                        Royal College of General Practitioners.

Contents

                                                                    Page

General Introduction: 1

           PART ONE : MODIFIED ESSAY QUESTIONS

1. A Postgraduate Exercise in Clinical Medicine
   and Primary Medical Care   11
   Answers   18
   Content Analysis   21

2. A Postgraduate Exercise in Neurology and
   Primary Medical Care   22
   Answers   31
   Content Analysis   36

3. A Postgraduate Exercise in Cardiology and
   Primary Medical Care   37
   Answers   45
   Content Analysis   51

4. A Postgraduate Exercise in Gastro-enterology
   and Primary Medical Care   52
   Answers   59
   Content Analysis   64

5. An Undergraduate Exercise in Psychiatry   65
   Answers   70
   Content Analysis   71

6. An Undergraduate Exercise in Microbiology   72
   Answers   76
   Content Analysis   78

7. An Undergraduate Exercise in Clinical Medicine   79
   Answers   87
   Content Analysis   91

8. A Preclinical Undergraduate Exercise in
   Human Behaviour   92
   Answers   99
   Content Analysis   101

9. A Preclinical Undergraduate Exercise in
   Human Behaviour   102
   Answers   106
   Content Analysis   107

10. A Preclinical Undergraduate Exercise in
    Human Behaviour   108
    Answers   112
    Content Analysis   114

11. An Exercise in Medicine and the Law   115
    Answers   121
    Content Analysis   123

12. A Multidisciplinary Exercise   124
    Answers   129
    Content Analysis   131

PART TWO : THE FUNCTION OF THE M.E.Q.

1. The M.E.Q. : Development, Construction and Uses   134

2. The M.E.Q. in Postgraduate Teaching and Learning 140

3. The M.E.Q. and Undergraduate Education   143

4. The M.E.Q. and the Student   147

REFERENCES   150

INDEX   151

General Introduction

This book consists of two parts which may be read independently.

Part I consists of a series of 12 exercises in diagnosis and patient care in the form of modified essay questions (M.E.Q.s) which the student can undertake at leisure. At the end of each M.E.Q., answers and educational feed-back are provided. In some instances, a marking schedule is provided : this should not be used out of context to assess the student's professional competence because in the examination situation in which the technique is used the M.E.Q. marks contribute only in part to a profile of performance. The marking schedule is included merely to illustrate how the serial structured essay question paper can be used to help to assess areas of professional competence not easily evaluated in other ways. Each M.E.Q. has been analysed in an attempt to show the kind of abilities being exercised : this analysis is included at the end of each exercise. The M.E.Q. can also be used by course organisers for group learning. The method can be guaranteed to generate considerable, even heated, debate which can enhance learning. Before the M.E.Q. is used in this way, teachers are advised to read the appropriate section in part II (chapter 2).

Part II deals with the development of the M.E.Q. and the possible uses of this learning/assessment device. It indicates how information about patients, readily available to many doctors (and especially general practitioners) can be organised to form original and, in our hands at least, extremely valuable teaching aids.

Medical education is a continuous process starting with undergraduate education, progressing through vocational training to continuing education. Throughout, the process is concerned with knowledge, skills, values and attitudes. One of the characteristics of the process is the difference in emphasis placed on these components at each phase. At the outset, for example, there is a body of factual knowledge to be assimilated, later comes the acquisition of particular skills, and all the time values and attitudes, which are dependant upon previous experience, among other variables, are being modified.

While much is known about the imparting of factual

1

knowledge, its comprehension, its recall and application, much less is known about skills and attitudes. The transmission of factual knowledge from teacher to students can be relatively straightforward, by lecture or text-book for example, and the class-room is a suitable setting; but the acquisition of skills, the appropriate modification of values and the development of professional attitudes are far more complex affairs. Such learning requires a great deal more consideration by both teachers and taught.

'With the enormous expansion in medical and scientific knowledge during the past thirty years or so, demands have inevitably come for the introduction of new subjects and the expansion of the old without any increase in the time allowed to complete the curriculum. As a result, medical courses have become so congested and excessively factual in content that their educational value is open to question.' - (Report of the Royal Commission on Medical Education, 1968.)

Yet, the criticism is even older than this -- well over half a century ago, Sir James Mackenzie was saying: 'There are two very distinct qualities of the human mind - memory and the power of reasoning. The earliest to be developed is that of memory and this can be cultivated with the greatest of ease. The power of reasoning is quite different, although no doubt memory takes a part. When we look at a great number of students, we discover that this power of memory is greatly developed in a few, but all our educational methods are devoted to its cultivation. Examinations are specifically contrived for the purpose of discriminating those who have the best memories and to them all the honours and prizes are given. Individuals who, on the contrary, possess more of the power of reasoning than their fellows receive no consideration.' (Wilson, 1926).

This failure to promote in 'psycho-motor' and 'affective' domains a similar development to that which has taken place in the 'cognitive' domain, is a characteristic especially of undergraduate medical education though postgraduate training is not immune; indeed, the failure is to be seen at its most grotesque in some present day contributions to the continuing education of experienced general practitioners.

Every doctor's personal experience teaches that skills and attitudes are acquired as much by practical as theoretical exercises. This frequently means some form of apprenticeship. The practical apprenticeship situation alone is, however, not enough. The apprentice can be taught to be either good or bad. Learning requires practical situations in which reactions can be monitored, analysed

2

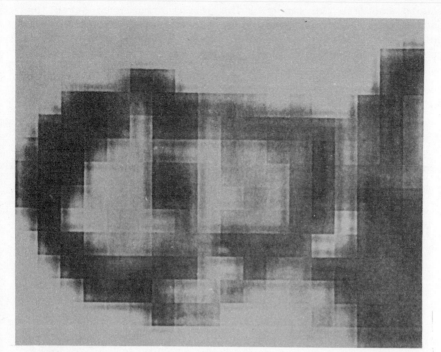

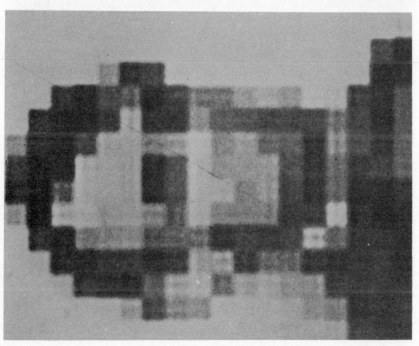

Figure 1

and when necessary corrected. These situations can also be used to evaluate the student. The serial structured situations described in this book provide a form of practical exercise that helps to teach some of the complex steps in diagnostic problem-solving and behaviour pattern recognition.

Two simple visual experiments demonstrate that recognition is a complex activity which involves several mental processes:-

1. Suppression of information. Look at Fig. 1 and then suppress some of the detail by looking with half closed lids, or at a distance or with insufficient light. The picture becomes more, not less, easily recognisable.

2. Pattern building

3. Association

4. Previous sensitisation

    a. Look at Fig. 2 which is a black rectangle and triangle

    b. now look at it again and think of the German leader who was largely responsible for World War II.

Pattern building and association enable us to see the rectangle and the triangle (Fig. 2) as the face of someone we know. For the process of recognition to be complete, the observer must have been sensitised to the faces of both Abe Lincoln and Adolf Hitler.

Let us now turn to the practical example of the medical student who must learn to recognise acute appendicitis in his patients.

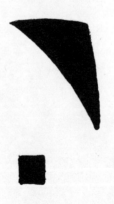

Figure 2

From books and lectures he learns much about the importance of different clinical features. He discovers that abdominal pain and right-sided tenderness are significant clinical pointers. A single vomit may be more significant than repeated vomits. If repeated vomiting is associated with repeated diarrhoea,then a diagnosis of acute gastroenteritis may be more likely than acute appendicitis. The student can thus be crudely sensitized to suppress, elaborate and associate the appropriate clinical evidence so that he can recognise the diagnostic pattern and predict likely events that must be prevented or managed. At this stage the process appears relatively simple and we often hear suggestions that a computer could handle the situation as well as or better than a doctor. Unfortunately in practice this relatively simple situation is greatly complicated by the patient's and doctor's subjective reactions. The patient will also suppress, elaborate and associate his own symptoms according to his previous experiences.

If we turn to a real life situation where the student is faced with a 10 year old boy complaining of abdominal pain of 12 hours duration brought up to him by two anxious parents, it is possible to list a few of the subjective influences that may cause the interacting patients and doctor to suppress or exaggerate symptoms:

1. The boy may be frightened and require time-consuming reassurance by the doctor before objective examination is possible.

2. The boy may be afraid of going into hospital and may distort subjective information about abdominal tenderness.

3. The boy may be too co-operative so that he says he is more tender than he really is.

4. The mother may be anxious and exaggerate some of the details of the boy's history because she wants the reassurance of hospital admission.

5. The mother may feel guilty about not having taken action sooner. She may therefore either minimize or exaggerate the boy's symptoms depending on what sort of person she is. She may even distort what has been done or said by a previous doctor.

6. There may have been a difference of opinion between father and mother about when the doctor should have been involved.

7. The student himself will be worried by his own inexperience and may be afraid of taking any responsibility for the diagnosis. He may therefore subconsciously emphasize those factors that justify hospital admission.

5

8. The student may be influenced against a diagnosis of appendicitis because there is an outbreak of gastroenteritis in the community, etc., etc.

The student must learn, assess and compensate for the effects of each of these subjective influences before he attempts to identify the true objective clinical pattern of the disease. Laziness, diffidence, insensitiveness, lack of empathy and experience in the student may all affect his ability to compensate in this way. We can now begin to understand why the attitudes of the doctor or student play such an important part in the practice of good clinical medicine.

In practice, the doctor deals with this complex situation by breaking it down. Each symptom or sign is isolated and considered in a circumscribed way before it is integrated to form part of the objective clinical picture. Thus, when assessing tenderness in the right iliac fossa, the doctor distracts the boy's attention to limit the process of association; when assessing the mother's story he takes into account his personal knowledge of the mother and so on, until he can build up the correct, objective, clinical pattern of the disease.

The structured clinical case history of the type described in this booklet can feed in enough circumscribed information about the patient as well as the disease to enable the student to consider and monitor the effect on clinical information of these distorting subjective influences.

The booklet is intended to encourage undergraduates and teachers to consider the learning process more widely. The techniques outlined are of course dependent to some extent on recall of factual knowledge from a wide range of disciplines, but they involve especially problem-framing and problem-solving and they can help to reveal attitudes. An interesting feature of the M.E.Q. is that unlike the multiple choice question it tests recognition as well as recall. This is significant because our ability to recall information is very closely linked to our attitudes and emotional involvement in any given situation or experience. A few simple personal examples illustrate this, eg: we can recognise many faces, places, books etc., when we are face to face with them but to recall a particular face, book, room etc., usually requires some emotional or attitudinal involvement. Such exercises are intended to increase the ability of the doctor to be more clinically effective in spite of scientifically inadequate data in his possession when he is forced to make decisions about problems his patients present. Fully developed, this is properly a postgraduate skill, but the foundations may be laid at an earlier stage. We believe that this should be a part of the scientific approach and incorporated into basic sciences courses.

There are several ways in which these objectives might be achieved, and this booklet is concerned with one of them - the Modified Essay Question. In recent years, the structured question has been used quite widely as an assessment device (Neale 1973). The M.E.Q. is a further stage in development, in which the dimension of time is built into the device. The M.E.Q. is, in effect, a serial structured question paper.

Students wishing to work through the M.E.Q.s are advised to do this *before* studying explanations, analyses of content and marking schedules. These have been placed at the end of each M.E.Q. deliberately because discussion of such matters beforehand reduces the impact of the problem-centred approach.

It is important that students wishing to obtain the most out of the exercises should write down their answers to each question immediately while they work through the M.E.Qs.

The answer layout of the questions is deliberate, and is necessary to avoid giving cues to answers to preceding questions.

We acknowledge out indebtedness especially to the Panel of Examiners of the Royal College of General Practitioners. The general practitioner tutors of the Departments of General Practice, Universities of Dundee and Newcastle upon Tyne have gone far beyond the call of duty in their efforts to develop the method.

M.E.Q. No. 2 and No. 3 have been used by the Royal College of General Practitioners in their examination for membership and M.E.Q. No. 4 is part of the postgraduate 'Check' programme of the Royal Australian College of General Practitioners. Figure 1 is reproduced by permission of Leon D. Harmon and the Scientific American. The E.C.G. is reproduced by kind permission of Dr J.A.R. Lawson. Mrs Carole Kent-Robinson was responsible for the onerous tasks of typing and collating the manuscript. To all the above our thanks are due.

PART ONE : MODIFIED ESSAY QUESTIONS

1. A Postgraduate Exercise in Clinical Medicine and Primary Medical Care

This M.E.Q. was designed primarily for use with post-graduates in a programme of continuing education.

An outline of answers is given at the end of this M.E.Q. (p.18) but the range of possible responses and the marking schedule are not supplied. An analysis of content and of abilities involved in responding to this M.E.Q. are set out on p.21.

The instructions which follow are an example of those which might be used in an examination. Readers wishing to try out the M.E.Qs are advised to write their answers on a separate sheet of paper.

Time allowed : 40 minutes.

INSTRUCTIONS

1. Please answer each of the 13 questions in sequence.
2. Answers should be brief. Do *not* give more answers than are requested.
3. Answers should be written in the space provided: if more room is required use the blank sheet opposite.
4. Please do not alter your answers after completing the whole M.E.Q.
5. Do *not* look through the book before you start.

Introduction

The Patient, Jim S., is an unmarried man born in 1923. He had rheumatic fever at the age of 9, when he spent several weeks in hospital. He served two years in the Army at the outbreak of the 1939 war, being discharged when routine examination revealed a cardiac murmur. He served his time as a joiner, but for the last 15 years he has been working as a talent scout for a football team.

You are the family doctor.

1. At the age of 32 he joins your N.H.S. list, when he consults you for the first time anxiously complaining of 'breathlessness'. On the limited information available so far, list three hypotheses to account for his presenting symptom:-

1.

2.

3.

2. It turns out that his visit to you has been precipitated by a friend who told him about a relation who had valvular heart disease and spoke in lurid terms about the accumulation of fluid and the hopelessness of the outlook. Your examination of his cardiovascular system leads you to the conclusion that he has both mitral and aortic disease, the predominant lesion being aortic incompetence. Give any three signs you might elicit to support your suspicion of aortic incompetence.

1.

2.

3.

3. Over the next few years, he remains in apparently good health not receiving any drugs. You have a record of his E.C.G. in his notes. Comment on (do not merely describe) his E.C.G. (Fig.3).

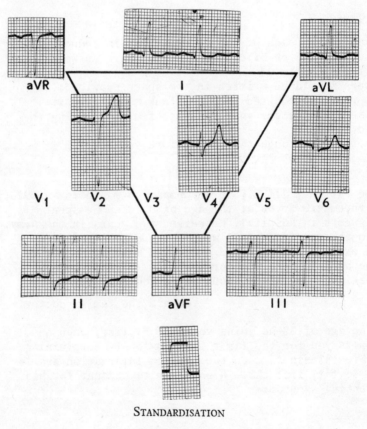

STANDARDISATION

Figure 3

4. In Spring 1967 a minor wave of influenza sweeps through
   your practice. On 24.4.67 he comes complaining of
   having had 'flu for a week -- by which he means malaise,
   vague joint pains and sweating. List three physical
   diagnoses you would consider and opposite each give
   two clinical features you might *elicit* to support that
   diagnosis.

DIAGNOSIS	SIGN/SYMPTOM

1.   i.

                                ii.

2.   i.

                                ii.

3.   i.

                                ii.

5. Following hospital admission for this episode, he settles down and continues at his work of talent-spotting, still on no drug therapy. Over the next three years he reports to your surgery on 11 occasions.

What does this information suggest?

6. In 1971 (he is now aged 48) he reports on 5 occasions in 2 months, each time with 'indigestion'. On the last occasion he reports that the medicines you have been giving him - Aludrox S.A. and Valium (diazepam) - have made no difference. What steps (if any) might you have already taken to help you form a hypothesis about the cause of this man's indigestion?

7. He now thinks he may have vomited up some blood though he couldn't be sure 'because it was rather brown-black material'. Select 2 of the most likely diagnoses you would not consider.

   1.

   2.

8. Barium studies reveal the presence of a probable neo-plastic mass in his stomach.

   Give 2 common sites in the stomach at which neoplastic changes may occur.

   1.

   2.

9. At laparotomy in October 1971 the neoplastic mass is confirmed and glands are found at the hilum of the spleen and along the lesser curvature. No metastases are seen, and so a retro-colic isoperistaltic partial gastrectomy is performed. Give 3 types of neoplasia which histological examination of the operation specimen might reveal.

   1.

   2.

   3.

10. The hospital discharge letter 11.10.71 states:
    *... Mr S. has made a satisfactory recovery and was
    discharged home on 10th October. The histological report
    confirmed the presence of neoplasia, but was rather more
    favourable than I had anticipated. The carcinoma
    permeated the gastric wall and mesentery, and whilst
    the peritoneal surface has been reached, only one lymph
    node appears involved.*

                                    Yours sincerely,

    What three important pieces of information have been
    omitted from this letter?

    1.

    2.

    3.

11. He apparently accepts the explanation that his operation
    was for the 'ulcer that caused his bleeding', and returns
    to work. He remains at work visiting you only occasionally
    for minor diarrhoea.

    Write in detail a prescription for the symptomatic
    treatment of his diarrhoea.

12. On 21.8.72 while consulting you for a repeat prescription,
    he says he has been very easily tired, has lost weight
    and is off his food, and draws your attention to a large
    lump about the size of a cherry just above and behind the
    left clavicle.

    What structure is likely to be involved?

    Why?

13. As you are examining him he says casually : 'I don't
    suppose it is really anything serious, is it?'
    Give in your own words your immediate response.

    List 3 factors governing that response:

    1.

    2.

    3.

END OF M.E.Q. 1

M.E.Q. 1 : RESPONSE GUIDE

Q 1   - Cardiac failure consequent upon rheumatic heart
        disease

      - Simple anxiety about the possibility of crippling
        heart disease (the actual reason in this instance)

      - Common respiratory diseases e.g. chronic bronchitis

      - Other answers are possible but less probable

Q 2   - Wide pulse pressure

      - Echoing diastolic murmur down left sternal margin

      - Enlarged left ventricle

      - Other answers acceptable if included in standard
        textbooks of medicine

Q 3   - Sinus rhythm

      - Possibly left ventricular hypertrophy

Q 4   - Influenza : Tracheitis
                     Little other abnormality at this stage

      - Subacute bacterial endocarditis : Embolic phenomena
                                          Constitutional upset
                                          Splenomegaly

      - Recurrence of rheumatic fever : Arthralgia
                                        Subcutaneous nodules
                                        Erythema marginatum

Q 5   - In NHS general practice 3 - 4 attendances per year is
        not significantly above that of an average person.
        This suggests that the patient has adjusted well to
        his condition and that his disability is minimal.

Q 6 - More information from physical examination (including specific mention of abdominal findings and, possibly, rectal examination)

- Stool examination for occult blood

- Barium meal

Q 7 - Peptic ulcer
- Gastric neoplasm

Q 8 - Greater curvature
- Prepyloric region

Q 9 - Mucus secreting cells
- Scirrhous carcinoma
- Epithelioid metaplasia

Q 10 - What the patient has been told
- What the relatives have been told
- What arrangement has been made for follow-up
- What on-going therapeutic regime is being followed

Q 11 - Some such response as :

R

Tab. codeine phos. 15mg.

30

Sig ī q.i.d.

is in order. The exercise in prescribing calls into play a variety of skills depending on experience, but for the trained general practitioner this would be mainly an exercise in recall with an element of clinical judgement.

Q 12 - Metastases to the left supraclavicular lymph node, because of the anatomy of the thoracid duct and lymphoid circulation.

Q 13 - Assess patient's reaction to what is a potentially fatal disease and in the light of this respond along the following lines:

- 'Well, what were your thoughts about this ...?'

or

- 'I'm sure you would want me to check this more fully ...'

In addition to the need to know more about the patient's reaction, responses by the doctor will be governed by other factors, for example:

- the need not to destroy hope

- the doctor's knowledge of the apparently hopeless prognosis

- the doctor's knowledge of the patient's strengths and those of the relatives

ANALYSIS OF M.E.Q. 1 : CONTENT AND SKILLS*

Content	Factual recall	Hypotheses Formation	Interpretation	Synthesis	Plan production	Application	Analysis	TOTAL
Clinical medicine	Q 2	Q1, 7		Q 4	Q 6			5
ECG			Q 3					1
General practice				Q 5				1
Pathology	Q8, 9							2
Patient management				Q10		Q13a)	Q13b)	3
Prescribing				Q11				1
Anatomy	Q12b)	Q12a)						2
	4	3	1	4	1	1	1	15

Before this M.E.Q. can be used for assessment, the weighting of the questions has to be agreed, depending on which abilities and which context are deemed to be important.

*The abilities listed in this table are not 'absolute'. They are subjective approximations and to some extent are related to the level of training of the participant (see Ch. 4). For each question only the most complex of a series of skills which might be employed is listed. The terminology is modified from Bloom's taxonomy (1956).

2. A Postgraduate Exercise in Neurology and Primary Medical Care

This question was originally designed to evaluate post-graduates working for the R.C.G.P. examination. The loading of marks is rather heavily in favour of doctors with neurological experience but otherwise gives a reasonable balance of knowledge and skills tested. It could easily be modified for final year students.

Time allowed : 60 minutes.

1. Mrs M., a previously fit, happily married 27 year old mother of two toddlers comes at a busy surgery to obtain treatment for her younger child's almost non-existent cold. As she leaves your consulting room she says, 'By the way doctor, if you're not too busy, I've been feeling very tired for the past two months'.

   a. What in your experience of general practice is the likely significance of Mrs M's statement, and

   b. What would you say to her?

   a.

   b.

2. Mrs M. tells you that she has had catarrh for years and that in the last two months she has had a headache, made worse by blowing her nose.

   What two *common* diagnoses would you consider to be most likely at this stage? Give three symptoms or signs that would help you to distinguish each diagnosis.

   a. Diagnosis (1)   b. Distinguishing symptoms or
                                              signs

                                    i.

                                   ii.

                                  iii.

Diagnosis (2)   Distinguishing symptoms or signs
                                i.

                               ii.

                              iii.

3. Two weeks later, Mrs M. attends accompanied by her husband,
   saying that her headaches are worse. The patient does not
   usually visit you with her husband. As the couple's
   relationship appears good and Mrs M. appears fit enough
   to come on her own you wonder why the husband has come.

   Give two possible reasons for the husband's presence which
   might influence your subsequent handling of this couple:

   1.

   ii.

   (You have now completed a quarter of this question paper.)

4. On detailed questioning, Mrs M. states that when she turns
   her eyes to her right she sees double, but if she turns
   her whole head to the right she can see things quite
   normally.

   What localising lesion does this suggest to you?

5. At this stage, give those diagnoses you might consider,
   listing them in order of probability:

   i.

   ii.

   iii.

   iv.

6. On this story, you strongly suspect the presence of an organic lesion in the central nervous system (CNS). You decide that a thorough examination of her cranial nerves and CNS is indicated. As you examine each cranial nerve in turn you look especially carefully for those signs that suggest early disease.

   a. Enumerate 4 findings that might suggest *early* involvement of the second cranial nerve.

   b. After each finding state the most likely condition that could cause this particular lesion.

   a. *Finding*   b. *Disease*

      i.

     ii.

    iii.

     iv.

(You have now completed half of this question paper.)

24

7. You perform a routine physical examination including blood pressure, urine and full C.N.S. examination. This appears to be entirely negative, so you arrange for a second opinion. As Mrs M. did not feel well enough to go to the hospital 15 miles away, the consultant sees Mrs M. at home. He thinks that the patient is suffering from a demyelinating disease and can be safely managed at home but says nothing to the patient himself. Mrs M. now says that apart from the headaches she feels fine.

Enumerate those things (in order of priority) that you feel it necessary to say to Mrs M. (or husband).

8. Two weeks later, Mrs M. is still complaining of her eye symptoms and headaches. Further examination of the patient's optic fundi reveals fresh findings that force you to the conclusion that the consultant's diagnosis may be incorrect.

a. Give three ophthalmoscopic findings in the fundi that are consistent with the history but incompatable with the diagnosis of demyelinating disease.

b. In each case give the diagnosis that is suggested by the finding.

a. *Ophthalmoscopic finding*   b. *Diagnosis suggested*

  i.

 ii.

iii.

9. You decide that full immediate investigation in hospital is indicated. You are anxious to maintain good relations with your medical consultant. No other neurological or second medical opinions are available. What would you say to him when you phone him to suggest that you would like him to reconsider his diagnosis:

    i. If he is a good clinician and a personal friend?

    ii. If he is touchy and liable to react to a colleague questioning his opinion?

(You have now completed three-quarters of this question paper.)

10. Four days later, after Mrs M. has been admitted to hospital, Mr M. comes to see you and asks you to certify him as unfit for work so that he can obtain money from social insurance while he is looking after the children. Mr M. openly says he is perfectly fit and that the note is only to enable him to get some money.

What action would you take to handle this problem?

11. About 7 days later Mrs B. a neighbour of Mrs M. tells you that Mrs M. died suddenly in hospital about one hour after having had what Mrs B. calls a 'lumbar punch'.

    a. What was the most likely cause of death?

    b. What was the probable lesion underlying Mrs M's case?

    What further actions would you take as a result of the neighbour's information?

    i.

   ii.

12. Three months after this, the patient's neighbour, Mrs. B. (aged 36) reports complaining of headaches, palpitation and dizzy spells. A routine physical examination including examination of fundi, urine and blood pressure reveals nothing abnormal apart from a regular pulse of 90 per minute and sweating hands.

    a. What differential diagnoses would you consider at this stage?

    b. If examination (including blood pressure and urine) were normal how would you manage the situation?

END OF M.E.Q. 2.

27

M.E.Q. 2 : RESPONSE GUIDE AND MARKING SCHEDULE

ANSWERS TO M.E.Q. 2.

Q 1. a. Any answer that suggests that the doctor
has realised that Mrs M's complaints are
of greater importance to her than her off-
hand manner suggests.   5

   b. Any statement that implies the doctor will
expand or investigage the patient's
complaints more fully either immediately
or in the near future.   5

                              Total possible   10

Q 2. The aim of this question is to discover the
general practitioner's knowledge of common
diseases: any mention of sinusitis obtained
with appropriate symptoms eg: discharge purulent
or blood-stained, morning headache worse on
movement, nasal obstruction or dullness on
trans-illumination.   6

Migraine or similar headache   2

Tension headache, depression, etc. also
allowed as one of the two alternatives   2

                              Total possible   8

Allergic rhinitis and hay fever are allowed
as headache is rare. Meningitis, space occupying
lesions, paroxysmal hypertension are not
allowed because these are not common causes of
headaches in a woman of this age. It is
considered inappropriate for the general
practitioner to investigate the patient for
these serious diseases on this evidence alone.

Q 3. Any answers that suggest two of the following:

   i. Husband or wife are more worried about the
illness than they care to admit openly   3

  ii. That the couple may wish in some way to
influence or put pressure on the doctor, eg:
want second opinion, etc.   3

31

iii. Patient feels that husband is in part
cause of her symptoms i.e. marital stress,
etc.   3

Total possible   6

Q 4. A straight clinical question. Mrs M. was seeing
double because of right external rectus weakness
when she turned her eyes to the right. By turning her whole head to the right she could re-
establish binocular vision.

Right external rectus weakness   3

Right 6th nerve palsy   4

Total possible   4

Q 5. Space occupying lesion or equivalent   4
Other diagnoses are not given marks as they
are all considered to be unlikely so that
in the practical situation they would not
have been seriously considered and would in
no way affect the doctor's actions.

Total possible   4

Q 6. This question aims to explore the doctor's
awareness that if you do not look for specific
physical findings you are unlikely to find
them. This section was eliminated as it was
considered that the question was too biassed
towards neurology. Any of the following would
have gained marks:

a. Blurred inner edge of   b. Space occupying
   disc   lesion or
   loss of cupping   retrobulbar neuritis
   pink disc
   choked disc   Multiple sclerosis
   papillitis or papill-   "   "
   oedema

   temporal pallor of disc

   Scotoma in optic fields   Space occupying
                                   lesion or multiple
                                   sclerosis
                                   Pituitary tumour

Total possible   ?

Q 7. This question aims to discover how the general
practitioner would handle the couple after only
one attack of multiple sclerosis when the diagnosis
had not been fully substantiated. The marking is
based on the assumption that there are certain
things a general practitioner must do and other
optional actions.

Any statement that makes it clear that the doctor
feels there is still uncertainty or doubt about
the ultimate diagnosis or outcome eg: full impli-
cation of consultant's diagnosis discussed with
husband only   4

Discussion about further pregnancies. (The patient
may be aware of outmoded medical opinion that
pregnancy may be contra-indicated).   4

Optimistic account of disease process   2

(Warnings to patient concerning future deter-
ioration, incontinence, paralysis, etc. are not
considered appropriate at this time)   __

                                    Total possible   10

Q 8. This question is marked on the assumption that
a general practitioner by this stage must consider
the possibility of symptoms being caused by a
space-occupying (and therefore a potential
treatable) disease.

a. Papilloedema   b. Space occupying lesion
   choked disc, etc   Cerebral tumour
   haemorrhages   aneurysm   6
   Exudates
                          Total possible   6

Q 9. This question is aimed at exploring the doctor's
tact. In fact it was too obvious and non-specific
to be selective. There were however many interesting
and amusing answers that gave considerable insight
into the different relationships between general
practitioners and consultants   6

                                    Total possible   6

Marks

Q 10. This question is intended to explore a
simple problem of administration. In fact
those general practitioners who took the
easy way out and gave a certificate as
requested failed to take any steps to help
the father as well. The lazy doctor was
thus penalised.

Refuse certificate (unless husband has
disability)   3
or Mental stress over wife and give
certificate stating this. Giving certificate
alone is not allowed   1

Telephone employer or social security,fix
money without certificate   3

Send nurse, home help, health visitor or
discuss help from neighbours   3

Children to day nursery   1

       Total possible   10

Q 11. a. Coning of medulla
  Herniation of brain-stem   3

 b. Space occupying lesion including cerebral
  tumour   3
  This question was inserted to penalise
  further anyone who had not considered
  space-occupying lesion. In fact it was
  almost entirely non-selective

 c. Telephone hospital or consultant to check
  facts   3
  Visit or contact husband to discuss case
  in light of facts or supervise arrangements
  for long term family care   3

       Total possible   12

Q 12. a. Anxiety state, tension state, anxiety
  neurosis, etc.   3

  Thyrotoxicosis started by shock of
  neighbour's death   3

 b. Discussion and explanation of situation
  or therapeutic listening (reassurance alone
  not allowed)   3

	Marks
Tranquillizers	1
See again, check later or keep under observation	2
Total possible	12

TOTAL POSSIBLE FOR WHOLE PAPER = 88

ANALYSIS OF M.E.Q. 2 : CONTENT AND SKILLS

CONTENT	FACTUAL RECALL	HYPOTHESES FORMATION	ANALYSIS	APPLICATION	SYNTHESIS	INTERPRETATION	PLAN PRODUCTION	TOTAL
Human behaviour		Q 3	Q 1a	Q 1b, 9				4
Clinical medicine		Q 2a, 12a			Q 2b	Q 4		4
Neurology	Q 6a, 8a, 11a	Q 5, 11b			Q 6b, 8b			7
Patient management							Q 7, 10, 11c, 12b	4
Special investigation								0
	3	5	1	2	3	1	4	19

3. A Postgraduate Exercise in Cardiology and Primary Medical Care

Post graduate - Originally used as evaluation for post-graduates working for the R.C.G.P. examination. This paper demonstrated the way in which the loading of marks affects the results of the evaluation.

Based on the responses of experienced General Practitioners, the marking schedule demonstrates how decisions have to be taken above the borderline answers. If this M.E.Q. were used for teaching purposes these points would generate discussion. The scatter of abilities and knowledge tested is reasonably wide.

Time allowed : 45 minutes.

In 1957 Mrs A., a slightly built woman aged 32, with two girls (aged 3 and 6), moves into your area and registers with your practice. She tells you that as a child she had rheumatism and valvular disease of the heart. (No adequate records are available.)

---

1. What further 4 questions would you have put to the patient to elaborate these two facts?

    1.

    2.

    3.

    4.

2. You learn that the valvular disease may have occurred at 5 years old and that she had raised blood pressure with both her pregnancies. She has reported because she is about to have a dental anaesthetic for removal of 10 teeth and is afraid she might still have raised blood pressure.

On examination you find pulse regular at 90, BP 150/90, a slight displacement of the apex beat to the left. One feature of auscultation of the heart suggests that she may have mitral stenosis.

List 3 sounds you might have heard that would suggest this diagnosis:

1.

2.

3.

3. Enumerate 4 main points you would make in reply to the patient's query about her fitness for general anaesthetic, and dental extraction assuming that she has never needed digitalis.

1.

2.

3.

4.

4. The patient takes a part-time job in your surgery but does not report any illness to you or your partners until 1964 (7 years later).

Give four reasons why she may not have reported any illness to you.

1.

2.

3.

4.

5. 23.7.64 - She reports that her last four periods have been heavier than normal and that her last period was 10 days ago. A vaginal examination reveals a mobile bulky uterus about the size of a 12 week gestation.

On 6.8.64 a Gonadotrophin test is negative

What 3 diagnoses would you consider most likely in this case and what action would you take?

1.

2.

3.

Action taken:

You have now completed half the M.E.Q.

6. If the patient had been pregnant list three problems you would need to discuss with the patient.

   1.

   2.

   3.

7. In autumn 1964 the patient is found to be pregnant (E.D.D. uncertain) and is booked for delivery in hospital. She is referred also to a physician who initially confirms your clinical cardiac findings.

   While you are awaiting the physician's report, she becomes suddenly breathless with cyanosis of the lips and clinical evidence of congestive heart failure. There is no cough, chest pain or fever.

   Discussion over the phone with the physician reveals that he now considers the patient to be suffering not from mitral stenosis, but from a congenital atrial septal defect of the heart.

   a. If this new diagnosis of atrial septal defect is correct, describe 3 radiological findings in such a case.

      1.

      2.

      3.

   b. Give not more than 3 possible causes for the onset of cyanosis.

      1.

      2.

      3.

8. On 27.3.65 she was delivered in hospital but went into acute heart failure just after delivery. For this reason she was not sterilised. She was kept on the Pill for 2 years until:

24.1.67 - she developed a severe continuous pain radiating down both arms especially the left. She is shocked, but there are no other fresh findings.

What are the two most likely causes of later acute incident?

1.

2.

9. On 14.2.67 on discharge from hospital, she comes to see you very angry because the hospital Physician Dr X 'has stopped her Pill'.

She says 'I was told by the Obstetricians two years ago that I must on no account stop taking the Pill and now Dr X tells me in front of the whole ward that I should never have been allowed to take the Pill; what does he know about the Pill anyway, he's a physician?'

Give two possible reasons for Mrs A's anger with Dr X.

1.

2.

How would you handle this situation?

10. Over the last 3 years Mrs A's cyanosis and symptoms of congestive failure have steadily increased. She now finds the care of her last child an increasing physical problem.

Apart from drug therapy, what steps would you take to support her?

END OF M.E.Q. 3

M.E.Q. 3 : RESPONSE GUIDE AND MARKING SCHEDULE

Total possible

1. MARKS FOR ONLY *THREE* OF THE POSSIBLE ANSWERS –

    1. Any questions that elaborated cardiac function and effect of valvular disease, dyspnoea, oedema, chest pain, etc.   4

    2. Any relation of cardiac function to pregnancy   6

    3. Queries developing an assessment of severity of original attack (attacks)
    Repeated attacks
    Length of time in bed or in hospital
    Previous treatment, etc.   2

       Allowed: dates of attacks of rheumatism and how treated
       Was surgery / valvotomy considered?

                                               Total possible   12

    NOT ALLOWED :

    for Answer 1 – Has she any symptoms now?
                    (Nature of symptoms not given)
                    Any residual disability?
                    (Nature not specified)

    for Answer 3 – 'What valve disease and when?'

2. Any *three sounds* heard given 3 marks :

    Presystolic murmur   3

    Diastolic murmur   3

    Accentuated second sound. Pulmonary   3

    Opening snap   3

    Third heard sound / Split second sound /
                            Pulmonary area   3

    Accentuated 1st sound (Mitral or apex)   3

    Apical systolic murmur of Mitral Incompetence   3

    Split Mitral 2nd sound   3

                                       Total possible   9

NOT ALLOWED :

Murmurs timing not specified
A diastolic murmur over aortic area
A loud aortic 2nd sound
Systolic murmur site unspecified
Diastolic + radiation to axilla
High pitch 2nd sound at apex
Accentuated apical 2nd sound
Diastolic Thrill in mitral area
A closing snap after 2nd sound

3. This question to be marked on only 2 of the possible
   answers :

	Total possible
1. She must have course of antibiotics	4
2. You may have to raise the question of hospital or at least a competent anaesthetist with dentist. No general anaesthetic in dental surgery. Doctor must inform the dentist of her history of rheumatic fever and valvular heart disease.	3
Total possible	7

NOT ALLOWED :

She might need a prophylactic cover of antibiotic.

In consultation with dental surgeon, depending on severity
of heart condition and general health, I might advise
operation to be carried out in two or more stages.

That *she* should inform the dentist or anaesthetist of the
facts (letter from general practitioner would be helpful).

4. ANY *FOUR* OF THE FOLLOWING GAIN MARKS :

1. May not have had any symptoms or she has been
   too busy to notice them   1

2. She may tend to minimise her disability
   because
   - mothers and cardiac patients often do
   - doctors appear to be too busy
   - she is chronically ill

- of the insidious onset
- of fear of neurosis
- comparison with other patients
  reassures her   1

3. Difficulty on adjusting to dual role of
   employer/doctor   1

4. May have gone privately elsewhere - not
   been our patient   1

5. Afraid to mention symptoms because afraid
   severe illness will stop her working
   - needs money
   - loves job
   - operation or hospital   1

6. May expect doctors to notice her symptoms
   automatically   1

7. Reluctance because other staff have access
   to her records   <u>1</u>

                               Total possible   4

5. a. ANY *THREE* OF THE FOLLOWING :

   Fibroids   3

   Pregnancy with false negative test
   (with or without mention of threatened
   or incomplete abortion)   4

   Dysfunctional uterine bleeding/
   Metropathia haemorrhagica   3

   Missed abortion (carneous mole)   3

   Endometriosis   1

   Carcinoma of body of uterus - uterine tumour   1

   NOT ALLOWED : Menorrhagia (Unqualified)

   b. WHAT ACTION WOULD YOU TAKE?

   Action taken - any of the following:

   - referral to obstetrician, cardiologist
     or physician
   - second opinion   3
   - probably dilation and currettage
   - repeat pregnancy test
                                                         ——

                               Total possible   13

47

6.   *Total possible*

ANY *THREE* OF THE FOLLOWING :

- confinement must be in a specialist Unit
  under a cardiologist in hospital   3

- hospital confinement with sterilisation
  after delivery   3

- hospital confinement with subsequent
  adequate contraceptive advice   3

- termination, or possibility of it
  Hazards of continuing pregnancy justify   3
  therapeutic abortion on medical grounds

- the need to obtain adequate rest during
  this pregnancy   3

- adequate care of the family (by Welfare
  Services, etc.)   3
                                                       ___
                                  Total possible   9

Note: Candidates lost out if they mention other
       'problems' as opposed to the 'courses of
       action' intended.

7. a. ANY *THREE* OF THE FOLLOWING :

   Enlarged right side of heart   2
   Enlarged right auricle or atrium

   Dilated pulmonary arteries   2
   or enlarged hilar shadows

   Hilar dance   2

   Pulmonary congestion or increased vascular
   markings   2

   Enlarged heart   1

   Small aortic knuckle   2

   NOT ALLOWED - Left ventricular enlargement, right
                 ventricular enlargement

48

b. ANY *THREE* OF THE FOLLOWING :

Reversal of shunt (Right to left)	2
Multiple minute pulmonary emboli or infarcts Pulmonary thrombosis	1
Endocarditis. Subacute endocarditis has supervened	1
Congestive heart failure / Decompensation Pulmonary oedema	1
Intercurrent chest infection	1

Total possible 10

NOT ALLOWED - Pneumothorax or onset of atrial fibrillation, peripheral stasis myocardial infacrt.

8. ANY *TWO* OF THE FOLLOWING :

Pulmonary infarct or embolus	3
Myocardial infarct or coronary thrombosis Coronary insufficiency or oedema	2
Thrombosis of veins of both upper extremities (Thrombo-embolism)	1
Thrombosis in pulmonary vessels	2

Total possible 5

NOT ALLOWED - Myocarditis

9. a. *ONLY TWO* OF THE POSSIBLE ANSWERS TO BE AWARDED MARKS :

Private matters were felt to have been made public	3
She had always been frightened by Pill and now discovers she was right	
or - Insecurity because the Pill has been stopped, with fear of pregnancy or altered marriage relationship	2

What would you say to Mrs A?

b. ALL OF THE FOLLOWING :

		Total possible
Accept the anger by understanding attitude		1
Explain reasons for physicians statement		1
Confirm that Dr X is right and Pill should be stopped now with or without discussion of other birth control methods		1
		—

Total possible   8

NOT ALLOWED : 'Reassure'

10. ALL OF THE FOLLOWING :

1. Entry to nurseries or nursery schools, play group, early school entry or other help with schooling of children   1

2. Home help service   1

3. Meals on wheels (or local authority laundry service)   1

4. Neighbours or relatives (including husband and daughters) help Baby minders   1

5. Transport to and from school   1

6. Discuss problem with children's department, i.e. children's officer, or School Medical Officer   1

7. Housing : downstairs bedroom or bungalow; essential needs on a single floor   1

8. Health Visitor (or District Nurse, or Social Worker)   1

9. Stop her doing part-time work. Refer to Social Security if financial difficulties   <u>1</u>

Total possible   9

NO MARKS FOR : Convalescent home for short spell Holidays for children.

ANALYSIS OF M.E.Q. 3 : CONTENT AND SKILLS

CONTENT	FACTUAL RECALL	HYPOTHESES FORMATION	SYNTHESIS	APPLICATION	PLAN PRODUCTION	TOTAL
Clinical medicine	Q 2	Q 8	Q 1			3
Patient management			Q 3		Q 10	2
Human behaviour		Q 4, 9a		Q 9b		3
Obstetrics		Q 5a	Q 6		Q 5b	3
Cardiology	Q 7a	Q 7b				2
Special investigations						0
	2	5	3	1	2	13

4. A Postgraduate Exercise in Gastro-enterology and Primary Medical Care

This question is for postgraduate students and demonstrates the M.E.Q. in the clinical problem-solving setting without introducing any patient variables. The question could be used to evaluate or teach consultants as well as general practitioners. The analysis of content shows the relatively limited area explored by this question (see page 64).

(By kind permission of the Royal Australian College of General Practitioners)

ONE MONDAY MORNING

INTRODUCTION

You are practising in an outer metropolitan area with good private hospital facilities and a public hospital five miles away. Adequate pathology and X-ray facilities are easily available to you. You are a member of a four man group and you have been on duty for the weekend. It is Monday morning and your day begins at 8.00 a.m. with a few home visits.

Case 1 Daisy Matthews

Firstly you visit Mrs Daisy Matthews aged 56, whom you saw 32 hours ago with an attack of severe unremitting epigastric pain which did not radiate. The pain had come on fairly quickly after she had returned from the local dance on Saturday night. Enquiry about what she had eaten revealed that she had had sandwiches and cream cakes for supper and a couple of beers. Subsequently, she had danced until 11.0 p.m. The pain came on just after getting home at 11.30 p.m. and you were called at midnight. She had vomited soon after the pain began and several times after that. She had had no similar pain previously, indeed, she had never had epigastric pain before. Her bowels were open normally earlier that day.

Examination revealed a plump woman of about 11 stone, of average height (5 ft. 7 in.) in obvious distress. She was pale, a little sweaty, and restless as she tried to get into a comfortable position. Her BP was 160/90, pulse 110 per minute, respiration 20 per minute and irregular, temperature 36.9°C; her heart was normal except for tachycardia, and her lungs were clear. Her abdomen was

52

generally moderately tender but more so in the epigastrium.
There was no rigidity but there was mild guarding in the
epigastrium. Bowel sounds, although infrequent, were
present. The extremities were normal. She could not pass
urine for you to examine. Because of the severity of the
pain, you gave her 100 mg of pethidine; 25 mg IV and 75 mg
IM, which resulted in the pain easing.

You called on Sunday morning and found that the pain
had gone. She had had a few 'twinges' during the night, but
had slept reasonably well. She had stopped vomiting two
hours after the injection and now felt 'washed out'. Her
abdomen was now soft with some residual epigastric tenderness. A specimen of urine passed that morning was examined
and found to be crystal clear with a negative test for
glucose, albumin, blood and bile, and the pH was 6.5 .

QUESTION 1

Your provisional diagnosis when you saw her first would
have been? (Name the one most likely diagnosis)

QUESTION 2

List the other likely diagnoses you would have considered.
(Name the three most likely differential diagnoses).

1.

2.

3.

QUESTION 3

Pethidine was used because (Select one or more):

A. It is an effective analgesic in this considion

B. It relieves spasm of the gastrointestinal and biliary
   tract musculature

C. It is less likely to cause spasm of the biliary tract
   musculature than morphia

D. It is less likely to cause nausea than morphia

When you arrive on Monday morning, Mrs Matthews says she is very glad to see you, because ever since about 3.00 a.m. she has been in pain again. The pain is in approximately the same place, perhaps a little more to the right than before, and is constant but not as severe as previously. She says she feels unwell, does not want her breakfast and feels nauseated, but she has not vomited.

QUESTION 4

On this history, what diagnosis would be uppermost in your mind? (Name one only)

QUESTION 5

On examination, what signs would you look for to support your diagnosis. (Name three most valuable signs)

1.

2.

3.

Examination reveals a rather flushed woman, BP 190/100, pulse 100 per minute, respiration 22 per minute, temperature 38.2°C; in some discomfort. Her heart is normal and the lungs are clear. Her abdomen exhibits epigastric tenderness extending under the right costal margin where there is some guarding. On deep inspiration the tenderness under the right costal margin is increased and there is mild rebound tenderness. Her urine is tested again and is completely normal.

QUESTION 6

The most likely diagnosis now is : (name one only).

QUESTION 7

What would you do now? (Name the three most important steps)

1.

2.

3.

QUESTION 8

The complications which you watch for are? (name three)

1.

2.

3.

END OF M.E.Q. 4

M.E.Q. 4 : RESPONSE GUIDE

QUESTION 1

On Mrs Matthew's history and examination findings and her progress the next day, the most likely diagnosis is cholelithiasis. The sudden onset of severe epigastric pain in a plump middle aged woman who has had no previous symptoms of this nature is very likely to be due to gall- stones. Common precipitating factors are dietary indis- cretions, and she had eaten some cream cakes at supper; and undue physical activity. One wonders whether her vigor- ous dancing may have been a precipitating factor.

The examination findings of obesity, obvious pain, sweating, pallor, tachycardia, normal temperature and epigastric tenderness all strengthen the diagnosis of biliary colic due to gallstones. The vomiting in this case is almost certainly due to the severity of the pain. Moreover, the good relief obtained by IV and IM pethidine and the fact that only minor recurrences of pain had occurred during Saturday night also support the diagnosis. The fact that vomiting continued for a couple of hours after the pethidine was given suggests that she may have been suffering from one of the side effects of pethidine, namely nausea and vomiting.

Reference 1, pp. 668-669   Reference 6, p. 134

QUESTION 2

Acute gastritis, myocardial infarction and perforated peptic ulcer would be three differential diagnoses that most people would consider. Staphylococcal food poisoning can come on within two hours of the ingestion of food containing the heat-stable enterotoxin of Straphylococcus aureus, and since this woman had cream cakes for supper, which are a common vehicle for straphylococci, this diagnosis is a possibility. However, the typical picture of this condition is one of 'collapse' with severe vomit- ing, epigastric pain, pallor, sweating and a 'shock-like' state with hypotension, extreme weakness and often diarrhoea. The patient is prostrate and tends to lie in a limp state rather than moving about as Mrs Matthews was. On the balance of the evidence therefore, food poisoning is less likely than biliary colic.

Myocardial infarction should always be considered in cases of severe epigastric pain but it is stated in the

history that there was no radiation and therefore she had
no chest pain, there was no clinical abnormality of the
heart except tachycardia, and the lungs were clear. Moreover, she had epigastric tenderness which is less likely
to be present in myocardial infarction than in biliary
colic. She was not hypotensive as one might expect in
myocardial infarction. Further, her restlessness is more
typical of biliary colic than of myocardial infarction.
The balance of evidence is against myocardial infarction.

Perforated peptic ulcer can give severe gastric pain of
sudden onset, but it is usually,but not always, associated
with marked guarding and rigidity, sometimes board-like.
There is also usually a past history suggestive of peptic
ulcer which this woman does not have. Moreover, patients
with perforated peptic ulcer tend to lie still rather
than move about, and it is usual for bowel sounds to be
absent. This diagnosis is thus less likely than the two
previously mentioned.

Renal colic is another possibility although the pain is
not typical. One would expect more laterally placed loin
pain with renal colic, with radiation to the groin. Moreover, it would not be common to have epigastric tenderness
with renal colic, but rather tenderness in the loin.
Another point against renal colic is the fact that the
urine was quite normal the next day.

Urinary tract infection is another diagnosis some may
think of, but the severity of the pain and its site, the
normality of the urine and the fact that the patient was
better the next day are all against this possibility.

Another less likely diagnosis is bowel obstruction, which
of course usually gives a colicky pain of increasing
severity, and there is usually some reason why this has
occurred. Furthermore, although it may be relieved by an
analgesic it is unlikely to have settled down so quickly.

Other much less likely diagnoses include acute pancreatitis
which occurs in alcoholics and hypertensives, and in which
the patient is likely to be more shocked than Mrs Matthews
was and exhibit much more abdominal tenderness guarding and
even rigidity. Acute porphyrinuria and diabetic keto-
acidosis are rare metabolic causes of epigastric pain, and
herpes zoster and pleurisy must always be remembered; but
in the case of Mrs Matthews these are very remote
possibilities.

Reference 1, pp. 668-669

QUESTION 3

A and C are correct. Pethidine effectively relieves the

pain of biliary colic in most instances. However, it does not relieve spasm of the gastrointestinal or biliary tract musculature; indeed the converse is true. However, it is less likely to cause spasm of the biliary tract musculature than is morphia and therefore is to be preferred.

According to Goodman and Gilman, (1970), and Laurence (1966), it is untrue that pethidine is less likely to cause nausea than morphia although this is a commonly held view. What is true however is that it is less likely to cause constipation than morphia and if taken continually this tendency to constipation diminishes.

Of some importance in the treatment of biliary disease is the fact that both pethidine and morphia can cause spasm of the sphincter of Oddi. Many clinicians will give an antispasmodic intravenously at the same time as pethidine in the treatment of biliary colic, and sometimes the antispasmodic alone is effective in relieving pain.

Reference 2, pp. 255-260   Reference 3, pp. 231-232

QUESTION 4

On Monday morning the situation has changed and Mrs Matthews now feels ill, anorexic, nauseated and has constant epigastric pain, although not as severe as previously. The first diagnosis to consider on this history is acute cholecystitis. On the story, scarcely any other diagnosis would fit, although cholangitis is a remote possibility. One would not expect it to have occurred so soon and one would expect to see jaundice, although it does fluctuate in this condition.

Reference 1, pp. 665-667

QUESTION 5

The three most valuable signs to support a diagnosis of acute cholecystitis would be a positive Murphy's sign which Mrs Matthews exhibits, guarding and possibly rigidity in the right upper quadrant, again a sign exhibited by our patient, and fever; Mrs Matthews has a temperature of 38.2°C. Thus she has three of the most important signs, which combined with her history would leave little doubt as to the diagnosis.

Reference 1, pp. 665-667   Reference 4, p. 351

QUESTION 6

The history and examination findings now point very
strongly to acute cholecystitis and this in fact was
the lady's diagnosis. The other possibilities mentioned
earlier have become increasingly less likely with the
development of her new symptoms. One might consider the
remote possibility of a very small leak from a perforated
peptic ulcer leading to local peritonitis, but with no
previous history of epigastric pain, an ulcer is most
unlikely. The fact that her urine is clear makes urinary
tract infection most unlikely.

Reference 1, pp. 665-667   Reference 4, p.351

QUESTION 7

There may be some debate as to what are the three most
important steps at this time but most clinicians would
agree that relief of pain, the commencement of antibiotics, and hospitalisation, if that is possible are
important early steps. IM pethidine would be a suitable
analgesic; again preferable to morphia because it has
less tendency to cause spasm in the biliary musculature.

Penicillin and streptomycin are not now favoured as much
as antibiotics with a broader spectrum of activity. Thus
the tetracyclines, ampicillin, erythromycin and
rifamide (Rifocin-M) are used currently. Ideally, the
antibiotic to which the commonly infecting organisms are
sensitive should be able to reach the infecting organisms
both by diffusion from the blood stream to the site of
inflammation and also by being secreted in high concentration in the bile. The tetracyclines and ampicillin are
active against most strains of bacteria which cause acute
cholecystitis namely Gram-negative bacilli of the E. coli
and related groups which are enteric in origin, Strep.
viridans and very rarely, Cl. welchii.

Tetracycline is the antibiotic most commonly used in a
dose of 250 mg 6 hourly by mouth or by IV injection in
the form of rolitetracycline 275 mg per day or IM rolitetracycline 350 mg per day. If tetracycline is contra-
indicated such as during pregnancy, ampicillin 500 mg
orally 6 hourly can be used.

Rifamide and erythromycin are active against Gram-positive
organisms and a range of Gram-negative organisms at the
concentrations reached in the biliary tract. Rifamide is
excreted almost exclusively through the bile and thus is
useful in the treatment of infections in the biliary tract.
However, rifamide depends upon satisfactory excretion via
the liver and thus in the case of complete biliary
obstruction, its concentration in the bile is not high

62

enough for this drug to be effective. Rifamide is unfortunately still very expensive.

The question of hospitalisation may be a controversial one, although most clinicians would prefer to have a case of acute cholecystitis under regular observation if this can possibly be arranged. Regular injections of analgesics and antibiotics are easier in hospital and should complications occur, they will be more quickly detected.

Surgery may have been listed as a possible step, but the question of surgery in acute cholecystitis is still a controversial one. Writing from the Mayo Clinic Ferris and Sterline consider that early surgical intervention is indicated for acute cholecystitis after the patient has been thoroughly evaluated and any concomitant medical problems corrected. They do not consider it a middle-of-the night procedure but rather one that can be carried out the following day. They consider that delaying operation for more than 72 - 96 hours increases the pre-operative complications, operative mortality and post-operative problems.

On the other hand many believe in the conservative management of acute cholecystitis and rely on antibiotics, analgesics, and intravenous fluids and gastric suction if necessary.

No doubt individual doctors have their own viewpoint, as do their consultants, so that one cannot be dogmatic either way on this subject.

Reference 7, p. 864; Reference 8, p. 156; Reference 1, pp. 665-667.

QUESTION 8

The complications which the clinician will watch for include empyema of the gallbladder, gangrene and perforation of the gallbladder leading to peritonitis, acute pancreatitis, ascending cholangitis and cholangio-hepatitis, and occasionally subphrenic abscess.

Empyema of the gallbladder would be indicated by an increase in the intensity of the patient's symptoms with increasing pain under the right costal margin, tenderness, guarding and rigidity; accompanied by fever, chills and toxicity. This, if it progresses, may result in gangrene of the gallbladder with perforation, which then gives signs of peritonitis. The other complications mentioned usually occur later and will not be described further here.

Reference 1, p. 667; Reference 4, p. 351.

63

REFERENCES

1. Davidson,S. Macleod,J. (1974) Eds. *Principles and Practice of Medicine*, Churchill Livingstone, Edinburgh.

2. Goodman, L.S., Gilman, A. (1970) *The Pharmacological Basis of Therapeutics*, 4th Edition, Macmillan, London.

3. Laurence, D.R. (1966) *Clinical Pharmacology*, 3rd Edition, Churchill, London.

4. Kupp, M.A., Chatton, M.J., Margen, S. (1971) *Current Diagnosis and Treatment*, 10th Edition, Large, California.

5. Netter, F.H. (1962) The Ciba Collection of Medical Illustrations, Vol 3, *Digestive System* Part II: Lower Digestive Tract, Ciba, New York.

6. Netter, F.H. (1964) *ibid.*, Vol 3, *Digestive System* Part II: Liver, Biliary Tract and Pancreas, Ciba, New York.

7. Ferris, D.O., Sterling, W.A. (1967) Surgery of the biliary tract *Surgical Clinics of North America* Vol. 47, No.4.

8. Tolhurst, J.C., Buckle, G., and Williams, S.W. (1972) *Chemotherapy with Antibiotics and Allied Drugs*. 3rd Edition. National Health and Medical Research Council, Canberra.

ANALYSIS OF M.E.Q. 4 : CONTENT AND SKILLS

Content	Factual Recall	Hypotheses formation	Synthesis	Plan production	TOTAL
Clinical medicine	Q 8	Q 1,2,4,5	Q 5		6
Therapeutics	Q 3				1
Patient management				Q 7	1
Human behaviour					0
	2	4	1	1	8

5. An Undergraduate Exercise in Psychiatry

This M.E.Q. has been used with medical students during a course in psychiatry.

1. Do *not* look through this booklet beforehand.

2. Answer question by question and do *not* turn back.

3. Indicate answers by putting a ring round the *one* response you judge to be most appropriate.

INTRODUCTION

Mr Emslie is a burly 60 year old warehouseman. He is a bachelor, living alone in the top flat of a modern multi-storey block, with all modern facilities, including under-floor heating. He consults you one Tuesday afternoon when the following dialogue takes place :

DOCTOR : 'Well, Mr Emslie, what can I do for you?'

Mr E. : 'It's these electric shocks coming through the floor (pause).'

1. In the light of the data so far presented would you say to the patient :

   A. 'This symptom is new to me'

   B. 'Did you consult an electrician?'

   C. 'Yes ...?'

   D. 'But that's unlikely, surely?'

   E. 'I've had several cases like this'.

2. So far, what seems most likely? He is :

   A. Misinterpreting normal stimuli ('illusions')

   B. In fact sustaining electric shocks

   C. Expressing sensations unrelated to reality (delusions)

   D. Deliberately inventing a story for personal gain (malingering).

3. *DR* : Through the floor of ...?

   Mr E : Of the house

   DR : Is it one room or every room?

   Mr E : Every room.

   You have in fact formulated a series of hypotheses.
   You now proceed to test them by eliciting more information. The responses 'of the house' and 'every room' :

   A. Make it less likely that he is experiencing real
      phenomena

   B. Exclude 'delusions'

   C. Add nothing significant.

4. Your next line of questioning is governed by :

   A. When?

   B. Where?

   C. Why?

   D. How?

5. *DR :* Why do you think this might happen?

   Mr E : Well, it's the people down below that's doing it.

   The patient has clearly expressed hostility to a third party ('the people down below'). You therefore :

   A. Remain impassive

   B. Refute the allegation as nonsense

   C. Agree with him

   D. Say nothing but draw your chair closer to him.

6. Your next line of enquiring is governed by your need to know more about :

   A. His physical health

   B. Possible drug therapy

   C. Habits regarding alcohol

   D. A possible systematised delusional state.

7. *DR :* So what did you do ...?

   Mr E : I went to the police and they said I was to see you and have my circulation checked.

   The information now suggests a diagnosis of

   A. Probable senile dementia

   B. Paranoid psychosis

   C. Depressive illness

   D. Anxiety state

   E. Psychopathy.

8. Bearing in mind that your waiting room is full, and that you have to finish consulting early to attend a postgraduate meeting, would you in fact examine the 'circulation'?

   A. Yes

   B. No

   C. Not now, but another time

9. Granted that physical examination gives no further positive clinical information, would you prescribe any drug for him?

   A. Yes

   B. No.

10. If you answered 'Yes', write your prescription here :

11. If you answered 'No', give two possible reasons for your decision:

    i.

    ii.

12. He now tells you that in 10 days time he is going down South on holiday for two weeks. This information will :

    A. Not materially affect management

    B. Cause you to increase his supply of drugs

    C. Decrease any urgency in the situation

    D. Determine the early involvement of specialist psychiatric help.

13. He flatly refuses psychiatric help, stating, 'It's not me, it's the people down below.'

    You will :

    A. Desist from attempts to get him to psychiatric help

    B. Admit him forthwith under certificates

    C. Attempt to get him to accept a domiciliary consultation.

14. Will you :

    A. Put him on the sick list?

    B. Keep him at work?

15. If you put him off work, indicate what you would write in the space for diagnosis on the Insurance Certificate:

16. If you keep him at work give two reasons to support your decision :

    i.

    ii.

END OF M.E.Q. 5

M.E.Q. 5 : RESPONSE GUIDE AND MARKING SCHEDULE

Q 1 :   A - 1   Q 2 :   A - 1   Q 3 :   A - 2
           B - 0   B - 1   B - 0
           C - 2   C - 2   C - 0
           D - 0   D - 0
           E - 1

Q 4 :   A - 1   Q 5 :   A - 1   Q 6 :   A - 1
           B - 1   B - 0   B - 1
           C - 2   C - 0   C - 1
           D - 2   D - 2   D - 2

Q 7 :   A - 1   Q 8 :   A - 2   Q 9 :   A - 2
           B - 2   B - 0   B - 1
           C - 1   C - 1
           D - 0
           E - 1

Q 10 : 3 marks for any appropriate scripts e.g:
placebo Tabs ascorbic acid 50 mg   20 - t.i.d.

Q 11 : Out of 3. Drug therapy does not help the condition.
Unnecessary risk of adverse drug reaction

Q 12 :   A - 0   Q 13:   A - 1   Q 14:   A - 1
           B - 0   B - 0   B - 1
           C - 0   C - 2
           D - 2

Q 15 : Diagnosis should be 'vague' e.g. 'Debility' Out of 2

Q 16 : Out of 2.
Work keeps him away from apparent focus of delusions
His earnings will be more than sickness benefit
He may lose his job, etc.

ANALYSIS OF M.E.Q. 5 : CONTENT AND SKILL

CONTENT	FACTUAL RECALL	HYPOTHESIS FORMATION	ANALYSIS	SYNTHESIS	JUDGEMENT	PLAN PRODUCTION	TOTAL
Medical interviewing					Q 1		1
Human behaviour		Q 2			Q 5		2
Psychiatry diagnosis				Q 7	Q 3, 4, 6		4
Psychiatry treatment					Q 13		1
Patient management				Q 16	Q8,11,12,14,15		6
Pharmacology					Q 9		1
Prescribing				Q 10			1
	0	1	0	3	12	0	16

6. An Undergraduate Exercise in Microbiology

This M.E.Q. has been used in a course in bacteriology for medical students during their first clinical year.

Time allowed : 30 minutes.

1. As family doctor, you are called to the house of Dr X, a middle-aged physician who ruefully confesses to feeling miserable. 10 days previously, while attending a medical congress in London he developed vague malaise and headache, followed next day by loose frequent stools, 3-4 per day. He dosed himself with diphenoxylate ('Lomotil') some samples of which he happened to have with him; this eased his griping abdominal discomfort.

   What pharmacological action is 'diphenoxylate' supposed to have?

2. Driving in easy stages, with appropriate stops, Dr X motored 400 miles home. He contrived to continue his work by resting up between times and dosing himself with codeine. His diarrhoea persisted, and he continued to feel out-of-sorts and so he is now forced to call you in.

   Give two aims which will govern your next questions :

   1.

   2.

3. Your general assessment shows him to look unwell. He is afebrile and his resting pulse is 80/min : physical examination reveals no significant information.

   To what end will your further investigations be carried out? (Do *not* at this stage list the investigations, merely indicate the hypotheses you might entertain on the limited information so far available.) Put down as many hypotheses as you wish.

4. Among the investigations you have requested, is the bacteriological examination of a stool specimen.

   a. What items from the information you have would you select to record in the box marked 'History' on the bacteriology form?

      'HISTORY'

   b. What examination(s) would you request your laboratory colleagues to carry out?

      'EXAMINATIONS REQUESTED'

5. In the bacteriology laboratory, the stool specimen undergoes certain procedures, one of which is culture in tetrathionate broth.

   Why is this medium used?

6. Next morning, several pale colonies are detected on both MacConkey and D.C.A. plates.

   Are these non-lactose fermenters (NLF) necessarily pathogenic?

                YES

                NO

7. If you answered *Yes* give one group of intestinal pathogens which you think might produce NLFs.

   If you answered *No* give one group of non-pathogenic organisms which you think might produce NLFs.

8. A pale colony has been subcultured into sugars, and peptone water, and inoculated on to urea, agar slopes and a purity plate. Next day the following information is available in the laboratory :

   (+ = acid and gas   - = no fermentation)
   Glucose +   Indole -ve
   Lactose -   Purity plate : pure growth of a
                                    non-lactose fermenter
   Mannite +
   Sucrose -

a. What is the next move the bacteriologist will make in the identification of the organism?

b. What kind of organism might now be suspected?

9. Serological reactions from the agar slope show agglutination with a polyvalent salmonella O; the organism is in specific phase (agglutination with H_1 and H_2). It reacts with group 'D' and 'g', showing that it is salmonella enteritidis.

To what clinical condition does infection with this organism give rise?

10. As the family doctor, you are phoned by the laboratory and told: 'It looks as if Dr X has infection with salmonella enteritidis sensitive to chloramphenicol, but resistant to ..... (and a long list of antibiotics follows).'

You have been treating your patient with mist kaolin and morph, and he says he is feeling a bit better.

Would you change your drug therapy in the light of the information from the bacteriology laboratory?

YES

NO

11. Give two reasons for your choice.

1.

2.

12. What factors govern your decision to allow Dr X to return to work?

What further action, if any, do you need to take?

END OF M.E.Q. 6

M.E.Q. 6 : RESPONSE GUIDE

Q 1 : - as a synthetic morphine derivative, it acts on
       smooth muscle of gut by blocking release of
       acetylcholine.

      - may produce dependence in long term.

      - drowsiness.

      - 'Lomotil' also contains atropine.

Q 2 : - to obtain more information about his present
       condition - duration of symptoms, other associated
       symptoms.

      - to obtain information about circumstances connected
       with onset (meals, or prevailing gastric-intestina-
       illness etc.)
      - to indicate empathy.

Q 3 : - food poisoning : bacterial
                          bacterial toxin
                          chemical
                          viral
      - dysentery : bacterial
                    other
      - acute appendicitis

Q 4 : HISTORY : - duration
                - presenting symptom
                - no antibiotic therapy given
                - if an infection, it has not been acquired
                  locally

      EXAMINATIONS : - culture for intestinal pathogens

Q 5 : - to inhibit the overgrowth of non-pathogenic coliform
       organisms

Q 6 : - No

7 : - Yes : - Shigella
            - Salmonella

    - No   : - Proteus
            - Pseudomonas

8 : a. Serological tests
    b. Salmonella

9 : - bacterial food poisoning

0 : - no

1 : - a. self-limiting condition :
        may prolong excretion of pathogens :

     b. risk of transfer resistance factors :
        toxicity of chloramphenicol :
        ? overgrowth of undesirable commensals.

2 : - a. his feelings of fitness
        (not bacteriological clearance not entirely
        symptom-free state)

     b. notify appropriate health authority, or other
        action indicating awareness of need to trace
        source.

ANALYSIS OF M.E.Q. 6 : CONTENT AND SKILLS

CONTENT	FACTUAL RECALL	HYPOTHESIS FORMATION	SYNTHESIS	ANALYSIS	JUDGEMENT	EVALUATION	TOTAL
Pharmacology	Q 1						1
Clinical medicine	Q 9	Q 2, 3		Q 4			4
Microbiology	Q5,6,7,8b		Q 8a				5
Therapeutics					Q 10	Q 11, 12	3
	6	2	1	1	1	2	13

7. An Undergraduate Exercise in Clinical Medicine

This M.E.Q. is aimed at medical students who have had clinical experience.

Time allowed : 30 minutes.

1. Mr T.H. an engineer aged 53 is a large man with a bluff hearty manner.

   He consults you, as a general practitioner, saying he has recently arrived in town and wants to register with you. 'By the way, doc', he says, 'I want some more of my pills - the "Cyclospasmol" or whatever they're called'.

   What is 'Cyclospasmol'? (Cyclandelate)

2. He has been taking this drug continuously for the past year for 'labyrinthitis', by which he means occasional episodes of dizziness and vomiting : from time to time he had attended the ENT out-patient clinic of a teaching hospital in another city.

   What considerations guide your information-gathering in the immediate next part of this consultation?

3. Two weeks after this consultation, he calls you to his house because he has been in bed for two days: "I feel a bit under the weather, doc : I suppose it's a touch of 'flu'."

   He has an irritative cough productive of only scanty mucoid spit. He gave up smoking on account of his 'labyrinthitis' a year ago, but had been accustomed to smoke 30 cigarettes a day before that.

   He is afebrile, has a slight inspiratory and expiratory wheeze and is a bit hoarse. There are no other signs on examination of his chest.

   Do you need further essential information at this stage to formulate a working hypothesis about his likely diagnosis and management?

   YES

   NO   (ring as appropriate)

4. If you answered *'YES'* list the essential information you feel you need. (List as many items as you feel necessary.)

   If you answered *'NO'* list your working hypotheses at this stage. (List as many probabilities as you wish.)

5. In addition to prescribing for him, you gave him an 'insurance certificate' excusing him from work for a week. His disability seems relatively mild and you confidently suggest that he should be fit to resume his work on the following Monday without further consultation. However, on the Monday, instead of returning to work he comes to see you. As he enters, you wonder why he should be consulting you at this particular time.

   Give three possible reasons for this consultation.

   1.

   2.

   3.

6. 'Your treatment's done no good, doc' he says, a bit huskily. 'I'm no better'.

   Clinical examination reveals no new findings : he still has scattered rhonchi in both lung fields.

   What do you see as appropriate next steps in his management?

7. Having referred him for a chest X-ray at the Mass Miniature Radiography Unit, you receive the following report:
'Right hilum and right paratracheal shadow: refer to chest clinic.'

That afternoon, before you have had time to take action, he puts in a house call. 'My cough is worse', he says aggressively, 'I feel bloody awful - and I've had a letter from the Clinic. I've to go and see them. Why? What is it, doc?'

List three factors governing your response to his question.

1.

2.

3.

8. His wife, a rather pretty woman who looks much younger than her husband is obviously very worried, but chatters away brightly in an effort to conceal her anxiety. 'Oh, you'll be all right, Tom' she says : then - turning to you for obvious reassurance - she adds, 'of course he will, won't he doctor?'

What response do you make to her?

9. Two days later, examination at the chest clinic confirms the clinical findings, and in addition a small firm nodule about the size of a pea is palpated in the right supraclavicular region.

What might be the significance of this clinical finding?

10. List 3 *investigations* most likely to confirm the hypothesis you have formed, and indicate which single test or procedure of the three you mention is most likely to give the greatest help in diagnosis and management.

1.

2.

3.

The one most helpful investigation :

11. Laryngoscopy reveals paralysis of the right vocal cord. You had considered the diagnosis of bronchogenic carcinoma as one possibility. Does paralysis of the right vocal cord occur more frequently or less frequently than paralysis of the left cord in bronchogenic carcinoma?

MORE FREQUENTLY

(Ring)

LESS FREQUENTLY

12. He proves to be a most difficult patient in hospital, and although he submits to biopsy of the supraclavicular lymph node, he flatly refuses to allow an arteriogram to be carried out.

Why might an arteriogram be indicated in this man's case?

13. Four weeks later, before you had a full report from hospital, Mrs T.H. 'phones telling you he's just been discharged home. If you were to visit him before you have a full report, what, if anything, might you aim to achieve by such a visit?

14. You find him very resentful of your medical and nursing colleagues, as he gives you a blow-by-blow account of his spell in hospital:
"They treat you as a bloody moron, they never tell you anything. They said it would only be a *small* operation and look, it's a 5 inch scar"(pointing to the biopsy site)."I was in for four weeks and they haven't found the cause of the trouble. If that happened in my work, I'd be thrown out of my job", etc. etc.

List three factors governing your handling of this situation.

1.

2.

3.

15. Next day, the discharge summary arrives listing strong
    evidence to support a firm diagnosis of inoperable
    bronchogenic carcinoma: the summary includes the biopsy
    report. What are the main histological features of a
    lymph node involved in metastatic bronchogenic carcinoma?

16. That afternoon he requests another house call because
    he has had a severe attack of coughing and breathless-
    ness. His wife opens the door, and obviously extremely
    agitated, asks you, as she leads you to him, : 'Why is
    his cough worse now, *after* he's been in hospital when
    he should be better?'

    What is the significance of this remark?

17. Next day, his wife 'phones again. He has been seen at
    the clinic that morning and she'll just call in 'for
    the new tablets the clinic doctor says he's to have
    with his X-ray treatment.'

    You have not yet heard from hospital about these tablets,
    but what are they likely to be?

18. You telephone the consultant, who confirms that Mr
    T.H. is to have prednisolone, 15 mg daily for the
    duration of his palliative deep X-ray therapy.

    Write the prescription which you will give to Mr T.H.

    R_X

19. You decide to take the opportunity of Mrs T.H's visit
    to discuss her husband's terminal care in his absence.
    What points will you aim to make in your discussion with
    Mrs T.H.?

END OF M.E.Q. 7

83

M.E.Q. 7 : RESPONSE GUIDE

Q 1 : - *vasodilator* with reputed selective *action on cerebral* blood flow which when improved is claimed to *improve mental function* in sufferers from *cerebral atherosclerosis*

Q 2 : - the need to know more about his disease
       - the need to know more about his disability
       - the need to know more about the treatment and management of his condition

Q 3 : - either, see question 4.

Q 4 : - YES - breathlessness or other chest or heart symptomology
             - proneness to winter cough
             - chest X-ray
             - lymphadenopathy
             - finger clubbing
             - did he stop smoking on *medical* advice?
             - job
             - previous general practitioner's views

       - NO - simple acute laryngitis / bronchitis
             - keep other possibilities in mind (bronchogenic carcinoma)

Q 5 : - existing disease or illness may have progressed (or not improved)
       - new disease has developed
       - social factor(s) may be operating : ie. need to have a few more days off work to qualify for benefit, or work problems

Q 6 : Investigation - X-ray chest
                    - E.S.R.

```
                        - peak flow meter
                        - laryngoscopy (possibly by consultant)
                        - previous records

        Therapeutic    - bronchodilator
                        - antibiotic
                        - keep off work

        Unqualified 'reassure' not allowed.



Q 7 : - my knowledge that he probably has serious disease
      - I don't know him very well
      - need to maintain initiative
      - my knowledge that he is a frightened man
      - need to avoid destroying hope, etc. etc.



Q 8 : - be non-committal
      - agree with need for investigation
      - full and early investigation - better prognosis
      - condition may be temporary and curable

      Reassurance alone is inappropriate.



Q 9 : - wide dissemination of disease (bronchial carcinoma)
      - poor prognosis : metastases
      - possibility of other lymph node disease eg. lympho-
        sarcoma
      - involvement from other local structure eg. thyroid,
        tuberculosis



Q 10 : - bronchoscopy
       - biopsy
       - sputum for malignant cells
       - one most helpful is biopsy



Q 11 : - less frequently



Q 12 : - pressure on subclavian artery
       - aneurysm of aorta or subclavian artery
```

Q 13 - rapport
  - hold initiative and trust
  - assessment of reaction by patient and wife to illness
  - future needs of support, continuity of drug treatment, etc.
  - his attitude to hospital treatment
  - allow him and wife to talk.

Q 14 - lack of factual information
  - he might have a cerebral secondary deposit
  - need to minimise apparently unjustified criticism of hospital colleagues.

Q 15 - replacement of normal lymph node architecture
  - by cells showing characteristics of the appropriate type of neoplasia (often 'oat' cell)
  - features of neoplasia (bizarre shapes and signs, pyknotic nucleus, etc. mitotic figures).

Q 16 - she is unaware of or has been unable to accept diagnosis or prognosis but may be affording you an opening to confirm her unexpressed fears.

Q 17 - steroids (prednisolone)
  - cytotoxic agents
  - antiemetic drug

Q 18 -

℞

Tabs prednisolone 5mg

(100)

Sig ÷ t.i.d.

89

Q 19 : - ensure she understands both nature of illness
and prognosis
- all is being done that is possible
- help will be forthcoming if cared for at home
- indicate willingness to help her - be accessable
- no pain
- because he is a difficult man discuss advisability
of his knowing
- need for discretion in answering her questions in
front of her husband.

ANALYSIS OF M.E.Q. 7 : CONTENT AND SKILLS

CONTENT	FACTUAL RECALL	HYPOTHESIS FORMATION	SYNTHESIS	JUDGEMENT	TOTAL
Pharmacology	Q 1				1
Clinical medicine	Q 9,10,11	Q 2, 4b	Q 3,4a,6,12		9
Human behaviour		Q 5	Q 14,16		3
Patient management			Q 13,19	Q 7, 8	4
Histology	Q 15				1
Therapeutics	Q 17				1
Prescribing	Q 18				1
	7	3	8	2	20

8. A Preclinical Undergraduate Exercise in Human Behaviour

Behavioural Sciences : Clinical Method

Time allowed : 30 minutes.

INTRODUCTION

Kenneth B. a very tall thin gangling 16 year old is the eldest of a family of three children (a brother 12 years and a sister 9 years). The father is a 45 year old clerical officer and mother is 43 years old, rather tense and very house proud. They live in a 4 apartment house on a fairly new Council housing estate.

You are the family doctor.

1. After school, Kenneth visits you towards the end of your afternoon consulting session. His record card shows he has not been to see you for 5 years.

   As he enters, unaccompanied, you wonder what sort of problems he might bring to you.

   In each of the three broad areas - physical, psychological and social - list 3 likely problems about which he might come and consult you.

   a. Physical
      (give 3 examples of   1.
      physical diseases common   2.
      at this time of life)   3.

   b. Psychological
      (give 3 examples of   1.
      psychological problems)   2.
                                  3.

   c. Social
      (give 3 examples of   1.
      social problems)   2.
                                  3.

2. Kenneth sits down and pointing to the lower chest says : 'It's this lump here'. What response do you make?

3. He had noticed a firm swelling at the lower end of his sternum, while in his bath the night before.

   Examination reveals a normal, though rather prominent xiphisternum.

   List three factors which might govern what you say to him.

   1.

   2.

   3.

You are now about one-third of the way through this assessment.

4. About a month later, Kenneth reports again, this time saying that he has a 'swelling down below'. This, it transpires, is a normal lower pole of the left epididymis and there is no other obvious abnormality in the genitalia.

   What would you say to him?

   Set down the actual words you might use.

5. He then asks if this could be V.D. At this stage, would you :

   a. firmly reassure that it is not V.D.

   b. indicate that you do not know

   c. ask why he raised this issue.

You are now half way through this assessment.

6. Give two reasons for your choice :

   1.

   2.

7. Mrs B., Kenneth's mother, reports the following week for 'the tablets for my nerves'. She usually attends your partner, and the last entry on her notes (3 weeks ago) reads : 'More anxiety symptoms – Repeat Valium 5 mg. t i d 60'. She says she's feeling better – not so tired, but would like to continue on the tablets for a bit longer. 'I feel they're helping me'.

Give three factors governing your response.

1.

2.

3.

8. At this point, your secretary rings through to remind you that you are already 10 minutes behind in your appointments.

As Mrs B. leaves she says casually : 'By the way, I'm a bit worried about Kenneth'.

What do you say to her?

Set down the actual words you might use in this situation.

You are now two-thirds of the way through this assessment.

9. It transpires that Kenneth has been absenting himself from school, associating himself with a tough gang from a nearby slum area, and is due to appear next day on a charge of petty thieving and malicious damage to property. His mother breaks down at this point, exclaiming in floods of tears : 'Neither his father nor I can do a thing with him'.

What is your immediate response to Mrs B's weeping?

10. She leaves apparently more composed, with a prescription for more Valium (say x 12). That night, Mr B. phones very aggressively demanding a house call because they've had a fearful row with Kenneth who has left the house : Mrs B. is hysterical, and has taken an unknown number of her tablets.

What is your plan of action?

11. List 4 broad emotional needs of adolescents in general-

1.

2.

3.

4.

END OF M.E.Q. 8

M.E.Q. 8 : RESPONSE GUIDE

ANSWERS TO M.E.Q. 8

Q 1 : a. - acne
         - trauma
         - epidermophytosis

      b. - anxiety : sexual function
         - feelings of inferiority : his size
         - 'lost' : problems of identity

      c. - conflict with family
         - stress : his job prospects
         - gangs, relations with peer groups.

Q 2 : - 'Tell me about it'.

Q 3 : - your knowledge that medically this is not a
         significant symptom
       - your appreciation that you are dealing with
         anxiety about a symptom - and not the symptom
       - your awareness that especially at this age group,
         any symptom may be merely an excuse to discuss a
         life situation.

Q 4 : - 'normal, don't worry about it' :
         'You seem to have a lot on your plate'
         or
         'It seems to me that things have been getting on
         top of you'.

Q 5 : - c.

Q 6 : - need to probe the whole situation after two vague
         offers
       - avoid limiting interview to VD issue

Q 7 : - need to meet patient's expectations
       - the fact that you are not her usual doctor

- your own views about prescribing psychotropic drugs
- your suspicions that Kenneth's problems are a part of the home situation, etc.

Q 8 : - 'Yes, I'd like to discuss this with you. Because I'm a bit caught up at the moment, could you come back - say this evening (tomorrow morning, etc.)'

Q 9 : - Remain silent, but indicate empathy non-verbally (lean forward, pat her arm, or some such.)

Q 10 : - accept aggression and indicate you will visit forth-with (Mr B.)
- visit to assess Mrs B's condition
- inform partner (Mrs B's usual doctor)
- possibly assist in finding Kenneth.

Q 11 : - need for defined limits
- need for freedom within these limits
- need to cope with anxiety
- need to be accepted (appreciated, loved).

ANALYSIS OF M.E.Q. 8 : CONTENT AND SKILLS

CONTENT	FACTUAL RECALL	HYPOTHESIS FORMATION	SYNTHESIS	JUDGEMENT	PLAN FORMATION	TOTAL
Human behaviour	Q 11	Q 1	Q 2, 8			4
Patient management			Q3,4,7,9		Q 10	5
Clinical medicine			Q 6	Q 5		2
	1	1	7	1	1	11

9. A Preclinical Undergraduate Exercise in Human Behaviour

Behavioural Sciences : Clinical Method

INTRODUCTION

Jim S. is a 39 year old garage mechanic, married to Dorothy, 38 : there are three children, boys of 15, 12 and 7. They live in the top flat (4th) of a modern corporation dwelling.

Jim has been back at work for 2 months apparently having made a full recovery from a severe myocardial infarction.

You are the family doctor and are called to the house at 3 p.m. one day because Jim has been brought home from work complaining of severe retrosternal pain-

1. Your physical examination makes you strongly suspect that he has sustained a further myocardial infarction. Apart from his history, list any 3 important clinical features you, as doctor of first contact, might expect to elicit at this stage on physical examination which would support your suspicions.

   1.

   2.

   3.

2. You intend to arrange Jim's urgent re-admission to hospital, and you telephone from the patient's house. While you are waiting to be put through to the hospital house physician, Dorothy (the patient's wife) shouts through 'Oh, Doctor, come quickly - I think he's dead!'

   The children have not yet returned from school and there is no one else in the house.

   List the next moves you would make and for each move give one or more reasons for it.

MOVE	REASONS

3. Immediate rapid clinical re-assessment now reveals Jim to be pulseless, cyanosed with pupils already beginning to dilate.

List the pros and cons of attempts to resuscitate this patient.

PROS	CONS

You are now one-third of the way through this assessment.

4. Your attempts at resuscitation are of no avail.

List the likely reactions of Dorothy to Jim's death.

a. immediately

b. within the next few weeks

c. after a year

5. The next door neighbour (a competent motherly woman, who is one of your patients) appears on the scene as you decide that Jim has in fact died.

List 3 ways in which you can channel her desire to help :

1.

2.

3.

You are now half way through this assessment.

6. List the pros and cons of prescribing any drug for
   Dorothy (Jim's widow) at this stage.

   PROS   *CONS*

7. Are you legally entitled to give a death certificate
   at this stage?

You are about two-thirds of the way through this assessment.

8. Would you ask Dorothy for permission for a post mortem
   examination?

   List reasons for and against your decision.

   FOR   *AGAINST*

9. List possible consequences Jim's sudden death might have
   on Dorothy's subsequent medical history.

10. Exactly one year later - to the day - Dorothy comes
    into your consulting room and suddenly bursts into
    tears. What is your reaction?

END OF M.E.Q. 9

M.E.Q. 9 : RESPONSE GUIDE

Q 1 : - Pallor; sweating; general appearance suggesting
        peripheral circulatory failure
      - Low pulse pressure; tachycardia; arrhythmias
        distended neck veins; basal crepitations. Signs
        suggesting heart involvement; pericardial friction
        rub.
      - The manner in which he describes his pain.
        (Clenched fist across praecordium : hands grasping
        praecordium : the moving restless elbow).

Q 2 : *MOVE*   *REASONS*

       Patient: Discontinue   He may in fact have 'died'
       phoning   and you will have to
       Hurry through to reassess   consider resuscitation

       Wife: Keep her in the   May need her help
       room   She may be too upset : in
       Keep her out of the room   the way

       Children: Arrange for   You don't want them burst-
       them to be met   ing in on you while you
                                   may be resuscitating

Q 3 : *PROS*   *CONS*

       Young man   This is the 2nd heart attack -
       Young family   you are less likely to be
       You are on the spot   successful
       Wife may expect you   You may revive him only to
       Society may expect you   have a chronic invalid on
       (Doctor's duty)   your hands

Q 4 : a. shock - complete failure to accept

       b. yearning - inability to accept fully

       c. acceptance

Q 5 : - comfort Dorothy
      - help with children
      - help with arrangements for funeral and contacting
        relatives, etc.

106

Q 6 : *PROS*

    May help with sleep
    Practical indication
    of Doctor's help
    Expectation of society
    Salves the doctor's
    conscience

CONS

    May merely add to patient's
    misery and confusion
    May be start of habituation
    May cause adverse drug
    reaction e.g. Overdose risk

Q 7 : - Yes

Q 8 : *FOR* - Confirm your diagnosis

    AGAINST - Add to Dorothy's misery. Unlikely to add
          to knowledge

Q 9 : - may make her more prone to depressive illness :
      suicide
    - may make her a higher user of medical services
    - may make her more susceptible to physical illness

Q 10 : - already prepared for anniversary exacerbation of
       grief
    - maintain understanding silence

ANALYSIS OF M.E.Q. 9 : CONTENT AND SKILLS

CONTENT	FACTUAL RECALL	SYNTHESIS	JUDGEMENT	TOTAL
Clinical medicine		Q 1		1
Patient management	Q 7	Q 2, 3, 5		4
Human behaviour	Q 9, 10	Q 4, 8		4
Therapeutics			Q 6	
	3	6	1	10

10. A Preclinical Undergraduate Exercise in Human Behaviour

Behavioural Sciences : Clinical Method

Time allowed : 30 minutes.

INTRODUCTION

Mrs McD is a thin anxious 24 year old, wife of a police constable, and mother of 2 children : Linda, a healthy looking 2 year old and David, 6 months. As her family doctor, you have supervised Mrs McD during the post natal period following David's uneventful birth.

1. Mrs McD consults you at the surgery with Linda (the 2 year old) saying: 'She's not walking right, doctor'.

   List 3 likely factors prompting Mrs McD's visit.

   1.

   2.

   3.

2. Mrs McD says that she has noticed that from the age of about one year when Linda started to walk, she seems to limp occasionally. Mrs McD is uncertain which let is affected.

   Of the many possibilities raised at this stage in your mind, give three *likely* physical conditions giving rise to Mrs McD's story and which would govern your further questioning.

   1.

   2.

   3.

3. In front of you lies Linda's past medical record. Select 3 pieces of information relevant to Mrs McD's visit which you would seek from Linda's notes.

    1.

    2.

    3.

You are now one-third way through this assessment.

4. Further questioning, perusal of notes, and physical examination lead you to the conclusion that Mrs McD appears to be worried about simple 'in-toeing' which you consider to be within the range of normal. What main points will you make to Mrs McD in your discussion with her? (List as many as you consider relevant.)

5. About 3 weeks later, Mrs McD brings (David (the second child now aged 7 months) for his 2nd triple antigen inoculation (against diptheria, pertussis and tetanus). As she leaves she says : 'By the way, I had Linda at the Welfare Clinic (ie. the Local Authority Child Welfare Clinic) the other day, and they said I was to bring her to you if she wasn't walking any better.'

    What message is Mrs McD trying to convey to you?

6. You visit and examine Linda at home the following day and find no physical abnormality of any kind.

    What do you say to Mrs McD?

7. Three weeks later, Mrs McD, apparently very agitated, enters your surgery with Linda saying : 'The Clinic doctor has just seen Linda and says you've to send her to a specialist'. She gives you a hand written note addressed to you in which the Clinic doctor writes: 'I examined the child today and can find no abnormality. Mrs McD seems unduly anxious - will you please see her?

    Would you comply with Mrs McD's demand forthwith?

                                                    YES
    Please ring your choice :
                                                    NO

You are now about two-thirds of the way through this assessment.

8. List factors governing your decision (record as many as you feel appropriate).

9. You go off on 3 week's holiday, and on your return you find a letter from your local paediatric consultant surgeon : it is dated a fortnight previously : 'I saw Linda at the Tuesday clinic when I was dismayed to find her with a characteristic limp due to congenital dislocation of the right hip. Her X-ray indicates that it is one of these hips that displace intermittently, but the fact that she's now walking must affect the ultimate prognosis. We shall get her in within the next week or so'.

   What significant pieces of information have been omitted from the letter?

10. List three of several important factors governing your next move.

   1.

   2.

   3.

11. List five behavioural phenomena which may be seen in families of handicapped children.

   1.

   2.

   3.

   4.

   5.

END OF M.E.Q. 10

M.E.Q. 10 : RESPONSE GUIDE

Q 1 : - Linda may not in fact 'be walking right' to such
        an extent as to require medical attention
      - Mrs McD may be unnecessarily anxious about a
        minor abnormality : paying undue heed to chance
        remarks by neighbours or to mass media
      - Mrs McD may be using this as an excuse to talk
        about her own problems

Q 2 : - injury (shoes too tight, etc)
      - congenital dislocation of hip
      - Polio, muscular dystrophy; variation of normal,
        etc.

Q 3 : - Frequent attender - decreases the weight you
        attach to Mrs McD's story
      - Vac. immunisation state : polio possible
      - any record of previous findings in locomotor system:
        for base line
      - birth injury

Q 4 : - normal phenomenon : allay anxiety
      - ask her why she was worried
      - indicate willingness to review situation
      - not to worry Linda
      - question of dealing with possible maternal
        insecurity

Q 5 : - she is still worried
      - she doubts your ability to handle the problem
      - she wants a third opinion
      - NO MARKS FOR second exam by you

Q 6 : 'I still can't find anything seriously amiss, but I
       understand your worry - what about getting an expert
       to help us?'
      - accept anxiety
      - willingness to have specialist help

Q 7 : Balance in favour of YES

Q 8 : Factors governing your decision to *REFER* :
       - there may be physical basis for symptoms
       - Mrs McD's anxiety needs to be dealt with
       - future relationship with family

       Factors governing your decision *NOT TO REFER* :
       - questioning your competence
       - possible waste of specialist's time

Q 9 : - what parents have been told
       - how they reacted
       - how the child got to the clinic

Q 10 : - need to discuss case with specialist colleague -
         get fully briefed
       - need to find out parents' reactions
       - need to be prepared to face litigation
       - welfare clinic informed
       - review the process

Q 11 : - limitation in family size
       - high prevalence of maladjustment to stress,
         broken homes
       - high prevalence of neurosis
       - prone to move house
       - prone to change general practitioner
       - spoiling by parents or sibs
       - rejection
       - tied to home

ANALYSIS OF M.E.Q. 10 : CONTENT AND SKILLS

CONTENT	FACTUAL RECALL	HYPOTHESIS FORMATION	SYNTHESIS	JUDGEMENT	APPLICATION	TOTAL
Human behaviour	Q 11	Q 1, 5				3
Paediatrics		Q 2				1
Patient management			Q3,4,8,9,10	Q 7	Q 6	7
	1	3	5	1	1	11

11. An Exercise in Medicine and the Law

This exercise is designed to introduce teaching of ethical and medico-legal principles by illustrating their application to a specific set of circumstances.

Time allowed : 30 minutes.

INTRODUCTION

Dr Green is the new assistant in a three doctor group partnership. Follow with him the situations presented in this document, and answer the questions *BRIEFLY.*

Mrs Valerie Smith is an 18 year old peroxide blonde who has been with the practice for one year since she moved into the area on her marriage.

She works full-time as a typist and has no children.

She consults Dr Green one day at the surgery saying : "It's that trouble down below again, doctor.'

1. By this, she means she has an irritating yellowish rather offensive vaginal discharge. 'It's been present for about 10 days now' - at this point she nervously falters.

   How might you elicit further appropriate information without breaking the line of the consultation?

   Write the actual words you might use:

2. Dr Green finds the following entry on her case record, dated about eight months previously:

   'Vaginal discharge, 7 days. Trichomonas vaginalis seen in wet preparation. Given Flagyl (Metronidazole) tabs. 21. To come again in 10 days'.

   There is no record of subsequent follow up.

   What is the causative factor of trichomonal vaginitis - how is it classified?

3. When Dr Green indicates he'd like to examine her, she resists, saying, 'Surely that won't be necessary? It's just the same as last time. Couldn't you give me the same tablets as before - they worked like a charm'; fluttering her mascara-ed eyelashes she adds, 'Besides, I've not come prepared.'

Of the various moves you might make, select the *one* you might choose in this situation.

4. At 1.0 a.m. two nights later, Dr Brown (one of the partners on call for the practice) is awakened by a telephone call. It's Mr Smith (Valerie's husband). In a rather slurred voice, and over background noises, which suggest a riotous party in progress at the Smiths, he aggressively demands an immediate house call because his wife's 'in agony' with the vaginal condition. He says: 'your pal's (meaning Dr Green) - your pal's treatment hasn't helped one bit'.

Is Dr Brown under a legal obligation to meet Mr Smith's demand?

5. Next day, Mr and Mrs Smith visit Dr Green in the surgery. 'I'll come to the point' says Mr Smith. "I'm not satisfied, doctor. First, Dolly here (jerking his thumb in Mrs Smith's direction) wasn't examined, then you - or your partner - refused to visit her. I'm not satisfied, and I want a specialist to see her.'

Dr Green, however, manages to get them to agree to allowing him an opportunity to carry out a vaginal examination.

All the other members of the practice staff are busy, but Dr Green decides to press on unaided with this important vaginal exam. Leaving Mr Smith in the consulting room he takes Mrs Smith through to the examination room and carries out a vaginal examination.

List two precautions Dr Green might take in arranging for the vaginal examination.

i.

ii.

6. Examination proves difficult. Insertion of the speculum is accompanied by screams and tears. Dr Green returns to the quiet of his consulting room bearing kidney basin. 'Well, old chap,' he says to Mr Smith, 'it's not serious after all: but, you really should be more careful'. And he exhibits a condom which has obviously been in the posterior fornix for some weeks and which he has just removed.

What important piece of information is missing from the Smith saga at this point?

7. Which *one* of the following contraceptive methods is most commonly used at present in the U.K.?

   a. the pill

   b. the sheath (condom)

   c. the dutch cap or diaphragm

   d. the intra-uterine contraceptive device

8. Mr Smith has turned pale - through clenched teeth he says slowly: 'But doctor, I've never used a sheath with Dolly'.

   Various medico-legal and moral issues affect the three persons mainly involved. List those which involve Dr. Green:

   Issues :

END OF M.E.Q. 11

M.E.Q. 11 : RESPONSE GUIDE

Q 1 : This question raises issues concerning interview
technique. Responses which indicate informed concern,
such as 'mmm, hmm ...' showing interest and waiting,
are more appropriate at this stage than embarking
on specific questioning about the apparent presenting
symptoms, or about other topics.

Q 2 : *Trichomonas vaginalis*, a flagellated protozoon, is
the appropriate response. Sexual intercourse as a
further factor is a suitable answer.

Q 3 : Encouragement to submit to examination is the most
appropriate move. If this move is unsuccessful, a
consensus view suggested that the issue should not
be pressed, and on the assumption that the symptoms
are due to a recurrence of the condition previously
recorded, drug treatment should be prescribed for
both the patient and the husband, with a request
that the patient should attend for follow up in 10
days.

Q 4 : If Dr Brown is satisfied from the information given
that no true emergency exists then he is NOT legally
bound to visit. The consensus view was that he
would be unwise to refuse to visit under the circumstances.

Q 5 : Precautions include:
- arranging for an appropriate chaperone
- wearing a protective glove
- ensuring the vaginal speculum is at an appropriate
temperature
- leaving the door ajar while the examination is
performed
- removing the husband from the room

Q 6 : No information has been given about the patient's
reaction to the findings. In her disturbed state
she may be assumed *not* to have appreciated what was
happening. She may not have given Dr Green permission
to divulge his findings to her husband.

Q 7 : In 1974, in the U.K. evidence suggests that the
sheath is still the commonest of the measures listed
with the oral contraceptive as a close second.

Q 8 : The important issue affecting Dr Green is breach
of confidentiality. He may have laid himself open
to a charge of assault on the patient. He may also
be cited as a witness in divorce proceedings raised
by the aggrieved Mr Smith.

ANALYSIS OF M.E.Q. 11 : CONTENT AND SKILLS.

	Factual knowledge	Judgement	Plan formation	Synthesis	
Behaviour		Q 1			1
Biology	Q 2				1
Patient management	(Q 5)		Q 3		1
Medicine and law	Q4, 5			(Q 9)	2
Medical ethics				Q7, 8	2
Contraception	Q 7				1
	4	1	1	2	8

12. A Multidisciplinary Exercise

This M.E.Q. has been used successfully in multidisciplinary course for social workers, health visitors, general practitioners and social work administrators.

Time allowed : 20 minutes.

INTRODUCTION

For the purposes of this exercise you are a general practitioner working from purpose-built premises with three partners and ancillary help : (receptionist, clerk and attached nursing staff and health visitor staff).

1. Mrs Betty B, a patient who is new to you and to the practice, comes with a little boy (Mark, aged 3) to consult you. She is rather plump, tidily dressed and she says 'It's his chest, doctor. I've been up the past 2 nights with his cough.'

   Indicate broadly what factors influence you most at this point in gathering information.

2. The medical history and physical examination indicate that Mark has no more than a minor common cold. This is not an uncommon situation in the experience of most general practitioners.

   Suggest some reasons why this happens.

3. About a month later, when it is your night on call, a neighbour phones asking you to visit Mrs B. in her multi-storey flat because Jimmy (4) another of Mrs B's children has spots. You are unable to obtain further information ('I'm only a neighbour').

   Indirect messages to the doctor requesting a house call have certain characteristics.

   Can you suggest two?

   i.

   ii.

4. On your way to another late call, you visit Mrs B. (about
   10.0 p.m.) when you find all Mrs B's 3 children fully
   dressed playing with their toys and watching TV.

   Jimmy's spots have features strongly suggesting flea-
   bites. What factors influence you in your management of
   this situation?

5. You note the over-heated, rather smelly atmosphere and
   the new furnishings (already rather battered) in Mrs B's
   top flat in a 23 multi-storey.

   Mothers in such buildings face several problems.

   Can you list any two?

   1.

   2.

6. Next morning, Mrs B. brings Jimmy to see you as you had
   suggested last night. Fuller examination confirms not
   only flea-bites but an infestation with head-lice as well.

   So far, in Mrs B's case there are now several indicators
   of a family with problems. Can you suggest any other
   'pointers' to a family in difficulties?

7. At this point, Mrs B says 'While I'm here doctor, could
   you give me a tonic, I'm so tired just now.'

   In this context, the likelihood of physical illness is
   outweighed by other possible causes for her request.

   List some working hypotheses to guide you in obtaining
   further information.

8. It transpires that not only is she behind with her
   'club' payments, but she has received a preliminary
   eviction notice from the Housing Department. Through
   tears she confesses to a bill of over £100 overdue
   to the Gas Board.

   Can you suggest possibilities of other social pathology
   inherent in this situation?

END OF M.E.Q. 12

M.E.Q. 12 : RESPONSE GUIDE

Q 1 : Factors include:
- the need to know more about the background of a
  family which is new to you
- the need to establish an appropriate relationship
  with the patient and the parent
- knowledge of prevailing morbidity in the district
- the time available for this consultation
- the hypotheses being entertained about what Mark
  could be suffering from

Q 2 : Patients may consult with a wide variety of
different motivations, among which are:
- desire by the patient for relief from unpleasant
  symptoms
- desire by the parent for relief from disturbed
  nights
- fear of possible future complications
- fear because of past experiences with others
  having the same symptoms
- genuine belief that medical science can cure the
  common cold
- desire to introduce a less socially acceptable
  topic (a 'cover story')

Q 3 : Indirect messages may become distorted, with
increasing degrees of urgency being injected en route.
The caller may resent being involved in someone else's
unpleasant affairs. Such calls usually provide
incomplete information, and it is sometimes difficult
to allot them an appropriate priority for action by
the primary health care team.

Q 4 : The information can be interpreted as indicating a
family which is failing to cope. Awareness of this
fact might help to modify the doctor's natural resent-
ment at such grossly inappropriate use of his services.

Such an episode is likely to be but *one* in a series
of future encounters. Consideration of how best to
manage the complexities of future relationships with

129

this family will temper the management of this
visit.

Q 5 : Mothers in new high-rise flats face many problems
      including:
      - anxieties about young children having to play out
        of sight and conflicts caused by having them
        constantly 'under their feet'
      - physical, social and sometimes cultural isolation
      - anxieties about vandalism, having to cope with
        lifts, and possibly new forms of heating, may add
        to worries about money (higher rents, increased
        transport and shopping costs).

Q 6 : Neighbours may occasionally report their anxieties
      to the doctor. The doctor and members of the health
      care team may fail to obtain answers when they knock.

      Failure of a child to make progress at school may
      be a pointer.

      Sometimes the family may simply vanish ('moonlight
      flitting').

Q 7 : While the possibilities of organic disease such as
      anaemia cannot be dismissed, the probabilities
      include :
      - anxiety about : marital relationships (including
                        sex)
                      : lack of money, and pressing
                        creditors
                      : difficulties with the law
      - loss of sense of direction and purpose to life,
        depressive illness

Q 8 : Throughout no information has been forthcoming about
      the husband. There is every likelihood that this is
      a 'broken family'. There may be undertones of
      alcoholism, prostitution, recidivism, etc.

ANALYSIS OF M.E.Q. 12 : CONTENT AND SKILLS

	Hypothesis formation	Plan formation	Factual recall	
Case history taking	Q 1			1
Behaviour	Q 2,3			2
Patient management		Q 4		1
Sociology/clinical medicine	(Q6), 7, 8		Q 5, 6	4
	5	1	2	8

PART TWO : THE FUNCTION OF THE M.E.Q.

1. The M.E.Q.:
Development, Construction and Uses

For over a century, the accepted measuring rod for a
sound undergraduate curriculum, at least in the United
Kingdom, has been the specific needs of general practice.
(Brotherston, 1971). Whether this was ever an appropriate
foundation is open to question, and it is only in recent
years that the concept has been seriously challenged.
(Royal Commission on Med. Ed. 1968). One of the effects
of this traditional educational aim has been to inhibit
postgraduate training and education in general practice
itself. 'After all', the general practitioner may ask,
'Why press on with education at postgraduate level in a
discipline which has been 'covered' by my undergraduate
days?' Yet, general practice is now seen to be a postgraduate discipline with its own characteristics.
(RCGP 1969). Now that the inhibitions are being over-
come, appropriate training for general practice is
forging ahead, and with it the need for assessment of
professional competence. The catalyst in these developments was the Royal College of General Practitioners,
which faced these new educational needs unhampered by
a traditional approach to the medical examination system.
A very great deal of time and effort was expended in
seeking solutions to new problems.

One of the problems was how to assess in a fair,
valid and reliable manner some of the professional
abilities of the family doctor, - abilities relevant
to all doctors, but especially relevant to the doctor of
first contact, the personal doctor, the doctor concerned
with continuity of care of the patient and his family
in sickness and in health. Clearly, no one test would be
likely to cover adequately all the requisite professional
attributes, and so there evolved the series of assessment procedures currently in use (R.C.G.P. 1972). The
objective assessment of the recall of factual information
over a wide range of disciplines was greatly facilitated
by the advent of the multiple choice question technique.
Yet, that method, in which possible answers are already
proposed did not lend itself to the assessment of
'creativity' ('pattern building') - the ability to
frame problems and to generate possible solutions : and
such skills lie at the very heart of all medicine -
especially primary medical care. Critical examination of
a range of other available tests confirmed the need to
develop a method more appropriate to the assessment of
such skills.

The idea of basing the technique on what actually occurred in an initial medical consultation and on the subsequent developments followed naturally. Such an approach was concerned with what in fact happened in the light of the information available at that stage - not necessarily what ought to have happened, or what the textbooks (if there were any) would say should happen.

In this way, it becomes possible to illustrate the inter-relation between behaviour presented by the patient (and behaviour of the doctor) and clinical medicine. In the hospital setting, such considerations tend to be obscured by the element of referral, because the hospital doctor is faced with giving a colleague an opinion as well as treating the patient, and the patient has not (usually) initiated the consultation. In addition, the necessity for immediate decision making is less pressing at hospital level. The decision to refer of itself may take the heat out of the situation because 'something is being done', but it can also make it difficult for hospital-based doctors to appreciate the importance of immediacy of decision making in medical care. The setting of general practice is thus particularly appropriate for developing methods of teaching and evaluation that use a problem-centred approach as exemplified by the modified essay question.

CONSTRUCTION

Selection of material

A case-history is selected by the originator of the project, from his personal experience and based on the records of the patient (and family) concerned - good detailed records are essential here. The main criterion for selection is suitability of the case to illustrate one or more components of the appropriate academic discipline - whether this be internal medicine, laboratory medicine, general practice, etc. For assessment purposes, the examiners of the R.C.G.P. selected general practice (R.C.G.P. 1971), but it is possible to use almost any setting, including the laboratory. Based on the factual experience of the doctor concerned, the development of the case is described in more detail, with sufficient information at each stage to reconstruct a series of circumscribed situations to which responses are invited. The responses may require an outline of action taken, a summary of the options open, a resume of factors likely to be operating, (including the feelings of patient and/or doctor), or simply the recall of factual information. It

is possible to determine beforehand the mix of abilities
to be assessed or exercised, and also to select the context
in which they are to be exhibited.

Unlike some problem solving tests, the development
of the situation in the M.E.Q. does not depend on the
options exercised by the respondent. This may lead to con-
flict between the thought process of the constructor and
those of the respondent, so it is convenient to reserve
on each sheet of paper a space for comment by the respondent if necessary. The sheets of paper, each bearing a
question, are then assembled in the appropriate time
sequence. The respondent is required to move only in one
direction (forward) through the M.E.Q., thus bringing to
bear the dimension of time in relation to the responses.
A complete example of an M.E.Q. is set out in Part I,
Example 1.

Validating the construction

To ensure that the M.E.Q. achieves what the originator
wishes, the assembled booklet is next subjected to comment
and criticism by a small group of doctors familiar with
the disciplines concerned, but who have not been involved
with the particular patient. It is at this stage that the
balance of the whole is reviewed. Whole questions may be
deleted, substituted or added, and the wording is carefully scrutinised and amended if necessary to eliminate
unintentional ambiguities.

Preparing the standard

The amended version is now duplicated and circularised
to a number of experienced and practising doctors, who are
invited to work through the M.E.Q. and record their responses. These answers are then collated, and for each
question a series of different responses is obtained. Sometimes their range is wide, but usually a consensus of
response is obtained over a narrower spectrum with answers
that may be appropriate, less appropriate - and occasionally a few which appear to the originator to be more
appropriate than the concensus.

It then becomes possible to classify responses
broadly in four groups: - the highly appropriate; the
appropriate; the less appropriate and those which are not
allowed. At this stage the originator confers with the
small panel : agreement is reached on the answers and
their weighting determined, the most appropriate receiving
the highest marks, the less appropriate responses being
given less marks, while inadmissible responses score no
marks. Part I, Examples 2 and 3.

The examination

Prior to sitting the test, candidates are advised *not* to read through the booklet beforehand. This is done not simply to preserve the surprise element of first contact medicine, but to prevent the distorting effect of hindsight. For example, a patient presents with sore throat to his family doctor : the candidate who lists acute leukaemia first when asked to record his hypothesis at this contact (on the limited information given) clearly indicates his lack of comprehension of the probabilities in general practice, even although the subsequent course of events proves this to be the correct diagnosis.

It is necessary at the outset to tell candidates the duration of the test and in addition to indicate the passage of time. This may be done by announcing the time at intervals during the test, and it has been found useful to incorporate into the booklet at appropriate places statements such as 'you have now completed one third (one half, etc) of the paper'. Candidates are also requested to resist the temptation to alter their answers when subsequent events make it clear that the response was incomplete or inappropriate.

Marking

When the completed booklets have been collected, the cover page on which is recorded the candidate's name is removed, and identification thereafter is by serial number, the same cypher appearing on each page of a given booklet. This minimises the 'halo or horn' effect which identification of individuals is known to exert occasionally on examiners.

Each question page is then separated and grouped with its kind from other candidates. The markers can thus concentrate their attention on a limited scope and by reference to the prepared schedule the allotting of marks becomes a relatively simple affair. Experience has shown that this cannot be totally comprehensive and allowance has to be made for the candidate who thinks up a highly appropriate response which has eluded the constructing team. It is desirable, therefore, that one of the markers will take responsibility to act as referee to resolve any difficulties immediately thrown up and for the group to be prepared at a late stage to amend the marking schedule. In the course of preparing the test, the 'index of difficulty' has already become apparent, and it is possible to implement the concept of a minimum pass level. However, one of the advantages of this assessment technique lies not so much in pass/fail information as in the light it may cast on areas of strength or weakness in a candidate's performance over a wider range of abilities than those concerned largely with recall of fact. It can usefully supplement information obtained from other more conventional assessment procedures, thereby helping to build up a 'profile of performance'. It is this overall profile which ultimately determines the pass/fail outcome.

The M.E.Q. is an effective teaching tool because it simulates the real life situation. The high degree of validity gives it great potential as an evaluation instrument.

The structured circumscribed format can be used effectively to decrease examiner variability - one of the well established problems of the traditional type essay question (Hartog and Rhodes 1935, Cox 1967).

The M.E.Q. can be used to reduce the unreliability of the traditional essay question in a number of ways.

1. *Content sampling :*

The short sectional format allows considerable spread of content to be tested. Content can be analysed (see part I) and deficiencies thereby identified can then be made good.

2. *Examiner variability :*

a. the circumscribed nature of each section allows a panel of examiners to predict all likely possible answers. A consensus of answers and the exact loading of marks can be agreed *before* the examination.

b. the structured nature of the questions allows accurate comparison of the candidates' answers with an agreed examiner concensus.

c. when an exceptional candidate gives an answer that has not been considered by the examiners it is possible to reconsider the examiner concensus view.

d. if pairs of examiners are used the variations of marking the itemised sectional answers can be easily checked and discussed.

Figure 3 shows how when using the itemised marking schedule on M.E.Q. 2 part 1 page   the correlations between pairs of examiners can be improved by checking the differences between these two sets of correlations.

We have some evidence to suggest that used in the ways described above the M.E.Q. method of assessment is more discriminant and reliable than the traditional essay question.

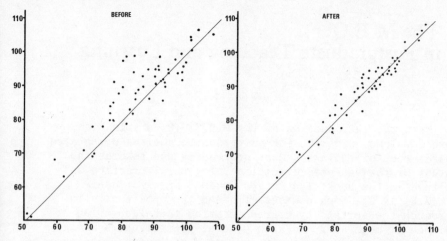

Figure 4. Correlation between pairs of examiners before and after checking the differences in marking of 58 papers.

Consumer response

Examinations are seldom regarded by examiners and candidates as 'fun'. Nevertheless, it has been our experience that assessment in this form has been the least unacceptable to most of 700 candidates experiencing the range of assessment methods employed in the examination for M.R.C.G.P. It was the enthusiasm of the doctors sitting the examination which was largely responsible for subsequent developments in applying the technique to teaching and learning.

From assessment to teaching

In developing and applying the M.E.Q. as an assessment method, what had been achieved? Briefly, it was this: the constructors had become less pre-occupied with the *content* of patient diagnosis and treatment and were more concerned with problems, with management, and with the *processes* involved. In other words, we had been forced to consider in a new light educational objectives. From there it was an obvious step to apply the technique to teaching and learning. In retrospect, of course, we were putting the cart before the horse, because in any educational process the first step must surely be a consideration of overall aims, specific objectives and then appropriate teaching and assessment methods, together with suitable feed-back mechanisms. Yet, at the time the M.E.Q. was evolving, the content and objectives had not been fully developed as they have subsequently become, nor was postgraduate training or undergraduate education in general practice so advanced.

139

2. The M.E.Q.
in Postgraduate Teaching and Learning

With the introduction of the M.R.C.G.P. examination there developed a demand for postgraduate courses orientated towards the College assessment procedures and towards the content of the academic discipline of general practice as outlined in the book: *The Future General Practitioner* (R.C.G.P. 1972). Such courses afforded the opportunity to introduce the serial structured question technique to an audience of motivated and keen general practitioners whose enthusiastic response clearly indicated their appreciation of this contribution from general practice to its own postgraduate needs. What began as a demonstration of an assessment technique soon developed into a heated debate, in which participants strongly defended their own favoured responses to given situations - and pointed out the short-comings of their colleagues. In short, a useful learning situation had been created. Early on, the leader learned of the need to minimise the risk of inducing in partici-pants unduly defensive reactions. One method of achieving this, and incidentally of disseminating and exchanging views more widely, is to ensure that in subsequent discussion of the M.E.Q. each participant does not go over his own completed paper. For such discussion group use, M.E.Q. papers are exchanged among participants, being identified by number only - this may be pre-printed on the book, in which case the participant has to note and remember that number if he wishes subsequently to retrieve his paper. Another method is for each participant to generate his own unique number; conveniently, the date of birth can be run together and linked with the initial for his surname (thus Dr Jones, born 10th March, 1927 would identify himself as 100327J).

METHODS OF PRESENTATION

The M.E.Q. can be used in a variety of ways in post-graduate teaching and learning. Most of the experience to date has been accumulated by its use as a focus for dis-cussion, but it has also been introduced as a self-audit device on a postal basis in Australia.

THE FOCUS FOR DISCUSSION

A fully prepared M.E.Q. which has been developed through the various stages outlined in the previous chapter, may be presented to the group of participants. They respond in the time allotted, and during a short break

the booklets are collected, shuffled and re-distributed.
The course reconvenes, and the leader goes through the
questions serially, listing responses already obtained from
the small group of experienced doctors (Ch. 1, p.122),
adding any additional and likely responses from individual
members of the course. He refers back to the group any
responses about which there is doubt. The ensuing discussion can help the originator of an erroneous view to
develop a new insight. Because it is done anonymously
and through the open discussion of a peer group the
learning experience becomes much less threatening than
would otherwise be the case; the risk of polarising or
antagonising weaker members is thereby diminished. 'Well,
in my view my answer is perfectly correct and you are
talking nonsense' becomes 'Look what this silly so-and-so
has written ...' Because the leader can 'distance' the
answers produced by the group of experienced general
practitioners whose standards can appear impossibly high
to some course members, the message can be got across
where - as usually happens - it is reinforced by the
majority view. 'Well, that's what that dedicated body of
practitioners felt about it, and judging by what I've
heard from most of you that's the way it is'. In such
ways it becomes possible to avoid the consensus of
mediocrity. If there is time, the participants may be
given the scores to be attached to the agreed groups of
responses, and thus each paper is marked by a member of
the peer group. While this allows rapid feed-back on an
individual basis, there is rarely time for collating
responses and the individual may be left with only a
hazy idea of his standing in the group. A modification
of this approach is to organise a team of helpers and
during a longer tea or coffee break to mark and collate
the results for presentation at the subsequent session.
Again, it is essential that individuals do not have
possession of their own papers while the feed-back
session is in progress if undue defensiveness is to be
avoided.

A further modification is to make use of an M.E.Q.
which has not been fully developed - or to take an M.E.Q.
which has in fact been fully developed but to present it
as if the group were to construct the responses as the
standard of reference. The steps followed are as set out
above, but *all* responses of the group are recorded on a
chalk board or written on acetate paper using an overhead
projector. The consensus modifies the range of responses,
but the task of the leader is much more difficult
because he has occasionally to exert a more authoritative
role if serious consensus error is to be avoided.

141

The upsurge of interest in postgraduate education has been associated with a renewal of interest in self-assessment. Some medical journals have incorporated multiple choice questions framed round the content of articles in their issues. A more ambitious project has been undertaken by the Centre for Education and Evaluation, Royal Australian College of General Practitioners. Every few weeks, a 'check programme' of self-assessment is sent to a list of subscribers. The programme incorporates various techniques - multiple choice questions, patient management problems, erasure problems and latterly, the M.E.Q. Once the participant in this postal course has committed himself to answering, the opportunity is afforded him of reading through a reasoned and consensus report against which he can evaluate his performance - and at the same time be stimulated to undertake further reading as required. An example is set out in Part I, Example 4.

More recently, this approach to medical education has been adopted by the postgraduate journal *Update* (McKnight, 1974).

3. The M.E.Q.
and Undergraduate Education

In view of the favourable reaction to the technique
in the postgraduate situation, it seemed reasonable to
attempt to apply it as a teaching/learning device to
undergraduate education. Yet, there were certain reser-
vations about extending its use in this way. Part of the
effectiveness of the M.E.Q. in postgraduate teaching lies
in the opportunities it affords participants to exercise
professional skills they already possess, though acquired
for the most part, the hard way - by experience. Would
undergraduates, whose maturity and experience are
necessarily restricted, find the method as useful?

EXPERIENCE WITH THE CLINICAL YEARS

The opportunity to find out occurred in 1971 when
a class of 5th year (2nd clinical year) students was
studying 'psychiatry in general practice', as part of
the psychiatry course.

By recording on sound tape patient interviews during
consulting sessions in general practice, it had been
possible shortly beforehand to capture and develop in
depth the presentation of a patient with paranoia. The
resulting M.E.Q. was then used in the context of the
psychiatry course; the objectives were to exercise problem-
framing and management skills as part of a demonstration
of the work of the first contact doctor and to re-inforce
specialist teaching about the disease complex 'paranoia'.
To heighten the impact, slides illustrating the patient
and where he lived were shown first and parts of the
tape-recording of the actual interview were played,
fitting in with the printed page in front of each member
of the class. To help the class members, some of the
questions were modified further to limit the open-
endedness. These were virtually multiple choice questions
in which the distractors were not 'false' in the usual
sense but were less appropriate to the given situation.
At the end of the M.E.Q. so adapted, a 'consumer type'
of rating schedule was incorporated in an attempt to
assess the acceptability of the exercise by the undergraduate participants. The class co-operated to the
full and the ensuing discussion threw up several
teaching points, such as the difference between the
clinic doctor's approach to the potentially hostile
patient ('remain impassive') and the personal physician
who has the future continuity of care to consider ('keep
quiet but indicate empathy by non-verbal cue'). By

applying the marking schedule (page 69) it was possible
to show quite quickly the discriminating nature of this
simple approach for this particular class (figure 5).
Analysis of the consumer response showed that all but 6
of the 55 felt that this was a useful teaching device,
and of those 6 only 2 students indicated that they did not
wish it to be developed further.

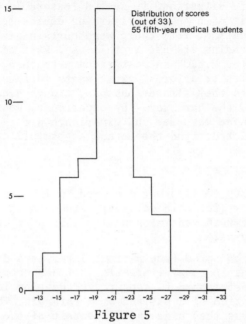

Figure 5

In the light of this response, the next logical
development was a joint specialist-general practice venture.
The opportunity for this presented in 1972 when a professional colleague developed food-poisoning. The clinical,
laboratory and community aspects of the episode seemed
appropriate contexts in which the M.E.Q. could be set.
Laboratory colleagues welcomed an invitation to collaborate
and the result is set out in Example 6. The level at which
this particular M.E.Q. is set is clearly deeper than most
general practice and hospital clinicians would accept as
realistic. This highlights one of the differences between
undergraduate education for the basic doctor and postgraduate training for the clinician. The response of the
class (4th year or 1st clinical year) was again enthusiastic
because of the learning in context.

A third development was to enlist the co-operation of
the *hospital clinical specialist.* Radical revision of the
curriculum of the early clinical years at the University
of Dundee afforded several opportunities in what is
called 'co-ordinated system teaching'. In the classroom,
students study the various systems (cardio-vascular,
respiratory, etc.) with contributions from various

specialist disciplines. This is complemented by clinical teaching in the hospital wards and, to a limited extent, in general practice. One means of bringing together the various strands in the classroom is afforded by the M.E.Q. which can help to provide a suitable perspective.

The clinician responsible for co-ordinating teaching of respiratory diseases agreed to select from his current hospital patients a case demonstrating several relevant teaching points. The case selected was a patient whose care was being shared by one of the general practitioner tutors of the Department of General Practice. The material thus gathered from the hospital point of view was augmented by a full discussion with the family doctor and primary health care team concerned, and the resulting M.E.Q. is set out in Example 7. This particular M.E.Q. has not at the time of writing been applied in undergraduate teaching, but it proved to be entirely acceptable at a postgraduate course for the M.R.C.G.P. (despite the exercise in factual recall of pathological histology!).

THE PRECLINICAL YEARS

Experience with the technique showed that it could be applied to undergraduate teaching in a variety of clinical disciplines. The inclusion of laboratory medicine had also been entirely acceptable to the medical student. Could the clinical setting be exploited as a medium for pre-clinical teaching? The ability of the M.E.Q. to pose problems of illness behaviour and clinical decision making suggested that the Behavioural Sciences course might be a suitable milieu in which to experiment. In 1972, the main educational thrust of the new department of General Practice at the University of Dundee was in a contribution ('Clinical method I') to the Behavioural Science Course. The opportunity was taken to apply the newly acquired experience to both teaching and course assessment.

From the wide range of possible topics, three were selected as suitable - adolescence, bereavement and the handicapped child. From past experience in general practice, augmented by appropriate case records, one patient (and family) was selected to illustrate features of each topic. The resulting M.E.Q. (and their marking schedules) are set out in Part I, Examples 8, 9, 10. The construction of these M.E.Q.s presented some additional difficulties because the level of background clinical knowledge likely to be possessed by a class of 19 year old students was unknown. Yet the clinical problems in the M.E.Q.s could not be ignored. As a compromise, a level little deeper than that of the intelligent layman was assumed and the marking schedule adjusted so that the clinical questions were not heavily weighted.

145

In each of the first three weeks of the course, the students were taken through the M.E.Q. *before* they had had the opportunity of much instruction in the Behavioural Sciences. After a suitable break, during which the booklets were collected the class reconvened. Before going over the details of each particular case, the teacher took the opportunity of delivering a mini-lecture attempting to put across salient points of the particular topic in general. Answers to the M.E.Q.s were then given, using specimens from the collected booklets and augmented by discussion with the class.

The fact of having responded to the M.E.Q. served several purposes. It gave each student a sense of personal involvement and a desire to know how his colleagues had fared. It also ensured that the class was on the same 'wave-length' as the tutor, and the motivation to learn was heightened. The M.E.Q. used in this way has been an acceptable and useful complement to other and more traditional teaching methods in the earlier years of medical education, and can introduce in context subjects like medical ethics (see M.E.Q. 11, Part I) which have hitherto received insufficient attention.

4. The M.E.Q.
and the Student

The nature of the abilities exercised has been
touched on in the foregoing chapters. In summarising the
situation it might be useful also to consider some of
the factors other than the M.E.Q. itself which influence
the nature of the learning experiences in the situations
described.

THE PARTICIPANT

One important extraneous factor is the maturity and
level of professional competence of the participant. The
information transmitted through the medium of the printed
word has to be *comprehended*; the situation indicated may
require *extrapolation* - blanks may have to be filled in
by imaginative thinking, though with the experienced or
trained doctor the filling-in may be accomplished by
factual *recall* ('Yes, I remember a situation in my
practice just like this ...'). On the other hand, the
problem-framing component for the untrained student may
have to be worked out from first principles or by
reference to the respondent's own life experience
('common sense') without a professional setting. Occasionally the information, e.g. deliberately transmitted in
the words of the patient, may require to be *translated*
into professional concepts and their implications worked
through. A more sophisticated method of exercising this
skill could be the presentation of clinical information
through slides or coloured pictures introduced at the
appropriate time along with the printed word. This presupposes that the participant already possesses the
necessary frame of reference.

Another ability exercised by the technique is that
of *analysis*. It is possible to introduce this in simple
form where the elements of the situation need to be
identified. In more complicated fashion, analysis of
relationships, especially human relationships and
analysis of organisational principles may be called into
play ('outline the main factors influencing your
response' to such-and-such a situation). Again the
response will be influenced by the previous experience
and life situation. It is at this level, especially and
again when *synthesis* is considered that the relationship
between attitudes and professional behaviour becomes
apparent. 'Attitude' in this sense is taken to mean 'an
idea charged with emotion which presupposes a class of
actions to a particular class of social situations'

(Triandis 1971). By this means the influences being brought
to bear on the participant - his attitude to his patients,
to his work and to his professional colleagues - begin to
be apparent. There is, of course, always the limitation
which applies to any reported response : there may be a
difference between what the respondent says he would do (or
think) and what he might actually do (or think) in the
actual situation. It has been our subjective impression
when using the M.E.Q. in conjunction with other assessment
procedures in the M.R.C.G.P. examination that there is a
good correlation between the attitudinal assessment so
revealed by the serial structured question and other assessment procedures purporting to be concerned with this group
of qualities (oral examinations, role play and simulation).
In general, the more experienced and better trained
candidates perform better in the M.E.Q. assessment that
the younger and untrained doctor - a contradistinction to
the M.E.Q. in which the scores of younger doctors tend to
be greater than those of the older more experienced
family doctors. The skills of synthesis, the ability to
produce a plan to solve problems or to derive a set of
abstract relations is at the core of much of patient
management. There may be cultural and even geographical
factors operating : for example, one M.E.Q. raised the
matter of dealing with a night call received by a general
practitioner when it was not his turn on duty for his
practice. There was a tendency for Scottish participants
to react by simply visiting the patient irrespective while
others indicated a variety of other means (passing the
call on to the appropriate doctor-on-call, attempting to
get the patient to accept a visit first thing next morning,
etc).

Closely related with the foregoing skills is the
question of evaluation, making judgements in terms of
internal evidence, and making judgements in terms of
external criteria. Again, while the experience of the
participant colours his responses the *nature* of the
ability exercised does not appear to be unduly influenced
by the respondent's state of training.

THE M.E.Q. AND THE PARTICIPANT

It has been pointed out in earlier chapters that the
M.E.Q. may be modified in various ways to suit the com-
petencies and educational level of a particular audience.
Thus, pre-clinical undergraduate students in a behavioural
science course require less emphasis on factual recall,
more on skills of synthesis and judgement, and a relatively
light clinical content. The clinical undergraduate student
will tolerate (and enjoy) a greater emphasis on factual
recall in clinical medicine. The postgraduate may need a

more balanced combination of the two, with problem-framing well to the fore.

POSSIBLE DEVELOPMENTS

The fact that the M.E.Q. has been employed to good effect with pre-clinical undergraduate *medical* students suggests that it might be an effective teaching device for judicious use in appropriate circumstances in the training of allied health professional workers. The authors have had limited but encouraging experience of using the M.E.Q. in this way at training courses for general practitioners and social workers, (eg: M.E.Q. 12, Part I).

The widespread interest in the problem oriented approach to medical records, P.O.M.R., (Weed, 1969) opens up new possibilities in medical education. Those teachers with clinical involvement with patients can use their records in the ward or in the consulting room as an adjunct to medical education. The P.O.M.R. approach could be helpful in constructing M.E.Q.s for use in the classroom. Such M.E.Q.s can themselves foster the problem oriented approach to medical care and assist in developing the skills of problem-framing, thereby preparing the ground during the undergraduate phase. The preparation of M.E.Q.s is properly a postgraduate exercise. This in itself is a very useful method of increasing awareness of educational objectives and the result is a convenient means whereby general practitioners can communicate with each other, commenting and criticising each other's responses. And such is at the very heart of improvements in patient care.

References

BLOOM, B.S. 1956 *Taxonomy of Educational Objectives* Handbook No.1 : Cognitive domain. Longmans, London.

BROTHERSTON, J.H.F. 1971 in *Medical History and Medical Care*. Ed. Gordon McLachlan and Thomas McKeowan, Nuffield Provincial Hospitals Trust, London.

COX, R. 1967 *Examinations higher education - survey of the Literature*. Universities quarterly 21 (3) 292.

HARTOG, P.J. and RHODES, E.C. 1935 *An examination of examinations* (New York: Columbia University. Teachers' College, International Institute. Examination Inquiry.) McMillan, London.

MCKNIGHT, J.E. 1974 *Clinical Challenge* Update, 8, 653.

NEALE, P.D. 1973 in *Assessment Techniques* by B. Hudson, Methven Educational Limited, London.

REPORT OF ROYAL COMMISSION ON MEDICAL EDUCATION (TODD REPORT). Cmnd 3569 1968 H.M.S.O. London.

ROYAL COLLEGE OF GENERAL PRACTITIONERS
1969 J.Roy.Coll.Gen.Practit. 18 358
1972 *ibid* 22 596
1971 *ibid* 21 373
1972 *The Future General Practitioner* B.M.A. London.

TRIANDIS, H.C. 1971 in *Attitude and Attitude Change* John Wiley and Sons Inc. London.

WEED, L.L. 1969 in *Medical Records, Medical Education and Patient Care*. Case Western Reserve University Press.

WILSON, R. MACNAIR 1926 in *The Beloved Physician*. John Murray, London.

Index

Analysis of M.E.Q. content
  MEQ 1 Clinical Medicine   21
  MEQ 2 Neurology   36
  MEQ 3 Cardiology   51
  MEQ 4 Gastro-enterology   64
  MEQ 5 Psychiatry   71
  MEQ 6 Microbiology   78
  MEQ 7 Clinical medicine   91
  MEQ 8 Adolescence   101
  MEQ 9 Bereavement   107
  MEQ 10 Handicapped child   114
  MEQ 11 Medicine and the
         law   123
  MEQ 12 Multi-disciplinary
         exercise   131
Attitudes   1,2,6,147,148

Construction   135
Consumer response   139,144,145

Examiner variability   138

Group work   140,141
Guide to using the book   1,7

Instructions to candidates 137

Marking   137
Marking schedule
  MEQ 3 Cardiology   45
  MEQ 5 Psychiatry   69
MEQ combined with lecture 146
Multi-disciplinary MEQ 12 124

Pattern building   4,134
Postgraduate learning
  Self-audit   140,142
  Group discussion   140

Postgraduate MEQ : examples
  Clinical medicine and
  primary care   11
  Neurology and primary
  care   22
  Cardiology and primary
  care   37
  Gastro-enterology and
  primary care   52
Problem definition
  Analytical approach   6
  Subjective influences   5

Recall of fact   1,2,6
Recognition   4
Reference standard   135
Relationship to POMR   149
Response guide
  MEQ 1 Clinical medicine 17
  MEQ 2 Neurology   29
  MEQ 3 Cardiology   43
  MEQ 4 Gastro-enterology 57
  MEQ 5 Psychiatry   69
  MEQ 6 Microbiology   75
  MEQ 7 Clinical medicine 85
  MEQ 8 Adolescence   97
  MEQ 9 Bereavement   105
  MEQ 10 Handicapped child 111
  MEQ 11 Medicine and the
         law   119
  MEQ 12 Multi-disciplin-
         ary exercise   127
Royal Australian College
of General Practitioners 7,52
                           142
Royal College of General
Practitioners   7,22,37,134

Skills   1,2,6,134,147

The setting of general
practice   135

Undergraduate learning
  Senior clinical students 143
  Junior students   145
Undergraduate MEQ : examples
  Psychiatry (MEQ 5)   65
  Microbiology (MEQ 6)   72
  Clinical medicine (MEQ 7) 79

Undergraduate MEQ : examples
  Human behaviour:
    adolescence (MEQ 8)   92
    bereavement (MEQ 9)   102
    handicapped child
            (MEQ 10)   108
  Medicine and the law
        (MEQ 11)   115

11/5/78

Difficulties

no data on reliability

insurmountable difficult as $\bar{c}$ scoring

Testmanship

Invalidity

? relationship to taxonomy.

poor for evaluation

good for teaching

152